THE COMPLETE ALTERNATIVE MEDICINE ENCYCLOPEDIA

700 Science Backed Treatments, with 100+ Diet Plans,

for 100+ Ailments A to Z

Welcome to *The Complete Alternative Medicine Encyclopedia* — your one-stop, science-backed guide to natural healing.

Inside this book, you'll find **over 700 remedies** for **100+ ailments**, from common conditions like colds and anxiety to more uncommon ones from A to Z. Every remedy is supported by **credible references** — books, medical journals, and clinical studies — so you're not just reading opinions, but proven, practical solutions.

Each ailment includes a **supportive dietary guide** with referenced suggestions to help your body heal from the inside out. And while some remedies appear under multiple conditions, that's because research shows their effectiveness across a wide range of issues.

This encyclopedia is intentionally written in **plain, simple language**. No complex jargon. No long-winded paragraphs. Just concise, easy-to-understand facts so **anyone can use it**—whether you're a complete beginner or already exploring alternative healing.

With over **700 scientific references** and remedies drawn from **doctors, researchers, and respected publications**, this is the most **comprehensive yet accessible** guide you'll ever need in natural and alternative medicine.

DISCLAIMER

This book is **not a substitute for professional medical advice**. Always consult with a licensed healthcare provider. These remedies are designed to support, not replace, the guidance of your doctor.

The information contained in this book is based on a wide range of **peer-reviewed sources, clinical studies, books, and journals**, and reflects an evidence-informed perspective on **alternative and complementary therapies**.

Alternative medicine refers to "a group of diverse medical and health care systems, practices, and products that are not generally considered part of conventional medicine."
— *National Center for Complementary and Integrative Health (NCCIH), U.S. Department of Health & Human Services*

In this book, the terms **"treatment"** or **"remedy"** are used to describe natural and holistic methods that may support or enhance overall health and well-being. These may include, but are not limited to:

- **Herbal medicine** (e.g., ginger, turmeric, ashwagandha)
- **Nutritional supplements** (e.g., vitamins, minerals, amino acids)
- **Functional foods and diets**
- **Mind-body practices** (e.g., meditation, breathwork, yoga)
- **Traditional therapies** (e.g., Ayurveda, Traditional Chinese Medicine)
- **Lifestyle adjustments** (e.g., sleep hygiene, hydration, stress reduction)

While many of these remedies are backed by scientific studies and have been shown to offer health benefits, they should be viewed as **complementary tools**, not cures. They are designed to support the body's natural healing processes and should be used **in conjunction with, not in place of, professional medical care**.

Table of Contents

ADHD (Attention-Deficit/Hyperactivity Disorder)

ADHD is a neurodevelopmental condition marked by inattention, hyperactivity, and impulsivity. While often managed with medication, natural and herbal remedies can support focus, calmness, and executive functioning by nourishing the brain and reducing overstimulation.

Herbal & Alternative Remedies for ADHD

1. **Omega-3 Fatty Acids (EPA/DHA)**

    - **What it does**: Supports brain development, reduces hyperactivity, and improves attention.

    - **How to use**: 1000–2000 mg/day of combined EPA/DHA (EPA-dominant ratio preferred).

    Reference:
    Bloch, M. H., & Qawasmi, A. (2011). *"Omega-3 fatty acid supplementation for the treatment of children with ADHD."* Journal of the American Academy of Child & Adolescent Psychiatry, 50(10), 991–1000.

2. **Zinc**

    - **What it does**: Essential for dopamine metabolism and brain signaling.

    - **How to use**: 15–30 mg/day with food.

    Reference:
    Arnold, L. E., et al. (2005). *"Zinc for ADHD: a review of the literature and meta-analysis."* BMC Psychiatry, 5(1), 9**Iron (only if deficient)**

    - **What it does**: Supports dopamine production and attention regulation.

    - **How to use**: 15–30 mg/day ferrous bisglycinate (check ferritin levels first).

    Reference:
    Konofal, E., et al. (2004). *"Iron deficiency in children with ADHD."* Archives of Pediatrics & Adolescent Medicine, 158(12), 1113–1115.

3. **Ginkgo Biloba**

- **What it does**: Improves blood flow to the brain and enhances memory and focus.

- **How to use**: 120–240 mg standardized extract/day.

Reference:
Salehi, B., et al. (2019). *"The therapeutic potential of Ginkgo biloba in neurological disorders."* Biomedicine & Pharmacotherapy, 109, 103–114

4. **Bacopa Monnieri**

- **What it does**: Supports memory, cognition, and stress reduction.

- **How to use**: 300–600 mg/day of standardized extract (20% bacosides).

Reference:
Kean, J. D., et al. (2016). *"Bacopa monnieri in cognitive performance."* Evidence-Based Complementary and Alternative Medicine, 2016, 5961031.

5. **-Theanine**

- **What it does**: Promotes calm focus by increasing alpha brain waves and reducing anxiety.

- **How to use**: 100–200 mg/day or in green tea.

Reference:
Lyon, M. R., et al. (2011). *"Randomized, controlled trial of L-theanine and green tea extract in children with ADHD."* Alternative Medicine Review, 16(4), 348–354.

6. **Rhodiola Rosea**

- **What it does**: Adaptogen that reduces mental fatigue and improves attention span.

- **How to use**: 200–400 mg/day standardized to 3% rosavins.

Reference:
Spasov, A. A., et al. (2000). *"Effect of Rhodiola rosea extract on attention and fatigue."* Phytomedicine, 7(2), 85–89.

Diet for ADHD Support

Recommended Diet Type: Brain-Boosting, Anti-Inflammatory Focus Support Diet

This diet is rich in omega-3s, antioxidants, and minerals that support neurotransmitter function, reduce inflammation, and stabilize mood and energy levels — all crucial for managing ADHD naturally.

Best Foods to Include

2. **Fatty fish** (sardines, salmon) – High in omega-3s for cognitive support
3. **Eggs** – Provide choline for brain development and memory
4. **Berries** – Packed with antioxidants that protect brain cells
5. **Leafy greens** – Support focus through magnesium and folate
6. **Pumpkin seeds and sunflower seeds** – Contain zinc, iron, and magnesium
7. **Avocados** – Provide healthy fats for brain cell structure
8. **Oats and quinoa** – Slow-digesting carbs for sustained energy
9. **Greek yogurt** – Rich in protein and probiotics for gut-brain balance
10. **Bananas and apples** – Provide steady glucose and fiber
11. **Green tea or matcha** – Natural L-theanine and mild caffeine boost

Why This Diet Works

- Provides key nutrients for **neurotransmitter balance** (dopamine, serotonin) Reduces **blood sugar spikes and crashes** that can worsen hyperactivity
- Enhances focus and memory through **brain-friendly fats and minerals**
- Minimizes inflammation, which can affect **brain function and behavior**

Scientific References for Diet & ADHD

1. **Millichap, J. G., & Yee, M. M. (2012)**. *"The diet factor in attention-deficit/hyperactivity disorder." Pediatrics, 129(2), 330–337.*
   ➤ Describes how elimination diets, omega-3s, and nutrient-rich foods reduce ADHD symptoms.

2. **Richardson, A. J., & Montgomery, P. (2005)**. *"The Oxford-Durham study: fatty acid supplementation in ADHD." Pediatrics, 115(5), 1360–1366.*
   ➤ Found significant improvement in attention and behavior with omega-3 supplementation.

3. **Stevens, L. J., et al. (2011)**. *"Nutrient deficiencies and ADHD." Alternative Medicine Review, 16(4), 284–295.*
   ➤ Reviews zinc, magnesium, and iron as key factors in managing ADHD symptoms naturally

Acid Reflux (GERD – Gastroesophageal Reflux Disease)

Acid reflux occurs when stomach acid backs up into the esophagus, causing heartburn, bloating, belching, and sometimes sore throat or chronic cough. GERD is the chronic form of this condition. Natural remedies focus on soothing the esophagus, improving digestion, and reducing acid overproduction without suppressing it completely.

Herbal & Alternative Remedies for Acid Reflux

1. **Deglycyrrhizinated Licorice (DGL) (*Glycyrrhiza glabra*)**

   - **What it does:** Coats and soothes the esophagus and stomach lining; helps repair mucosa.

   - **How to use:** 380 mg chewable tablets 20 minutes before meals, 2–3x/day.

   Reference:
   Morgan, A. G., et al. (1982). *"Comparison of DGL with cimetidine for healing ulcers."* BMJ, 284(6314), 1822.

2. **Slippery Elm (*Ulmus rubra*)**

   - **What it does:** Rich in mucilage; forms a protective coating in the throat and stomach.

   - **How to use:** 1 tsp powder in warm water after meals and before bed.

   Reference:
   Yarnell, E., & Abascal, K. (2004). *"Demulcents and mucilage in gastroprotection."* Alternative & Complementary Therapies, 10(5), 270–274.

3. **Aloe Vera Juice (Inner Leaf, Decolorized)**

   - **What it does:** Soothes and heals irritated esophageal lining.

   - **How to use:** ¼–½ cup of unsweetened aloe vera juice before meals.

   Reference:
   Langmead, L., et al. (2004). *"Oral aloe vera in gastrointestinal inflammation."* Alimentary Pharmacology & Therapeutics, 19(7), 739–747.

4. **Chamomile Tea (*Matricaria recutita*)**

- **What it does**: Calms digestive muscles, reduces acid production, and soothes irritation.

- **How to use**: 1–2 cups/day, ideally between meals.

Reference:
McKay, D. L., & Blumberg, J. B. (2006). *"Chamomile tea's role in soothing GI discomfort."* Phytotherapy Research, 20(7), 519–530.

5. **Apple Cider Vinegar (for low stomach acid cases)**

- **What it does**: Helps digestion by increasing stomach acid in cases of hypochlorhydria.

- **How to use**: 1 tsp in ½ cup warm water before meals (avoid during active heartburn).

Reference:
Johnston, C. S., et al. (2004). *"Vinegar improves insulin sensitivity; aids digestion."* Diabetes Care, 27(1), 281–282.

6. **Probiotics**

- **What it does**: Balances gut bacteria, improves digestion, and may reduce reflux symptoms.

- **How to use**: 10–30 billion CFUs/day of multi-strain probiotic.

Reference:
Riezzo, G., et al. (2000). *"Probiotic lactobacilli in GERD."* Journal of Clinical Gastroenterology, 31(2), 150–153.

7. **Marshmallow Root (*Althaea officinalis*)**

- **What it does**: Demulcent; protects mucous membranes and reduces acid irritation.

- **How to use**: Cold infusion (steep 1 tbsp overnight in cold water); sip throughout the day.

Reference:
PDR for Herbal Medicines (4th ed.), Thomson Reuters.

Diet for Acid Reflux Support

Recommended Diet Type: Low-Acid, Mucosa-Soothing, Alkaline-Supportive Digestive Diet

This diet avoids common reflux triggers while focusing on anti-inflammatory, alkaline-forming, and gut-soothing foods that help reduce symptoms and promote healing.

Best Foods to Include

1. **Bananas and melons** – Low-acid fruits that soothe the stomach
2. **Oats and brown rice** – Fiber-rich, low-fat carbs that don't trigger reflux
3. **Ginger** – Natural anti-inflammatory and digestion aid
4. **Leafy greens and cucumbers** – Alkaline and cooling for digestive tissues
5. **Sweet potatoes and squash** – Gentle on digestion and non-acidic
6. **Almonds** – Contain healthy fats and may reduce stomach acid
7. **Non-citrus smoothies** – Cool, gentle on the esophagus
8. **Licorice and chamomile tea** – Reduce inflammation and coat the gut
9. **Fermented foods (if tolerated)** – Support a healthy microbiome
10. **Filtered water** – Helps dilute acid and flush digestive tract

Why This Diet Works

- Reduces intake of **acidic, spicy, and high-fat foods** that weaken the lower esophageal sphincter

- Promotes **healing of esophageal tissues** with mucilaginous herbs and gentle foods

- Supports **proper digestion** to prevent pressure build-up in the stomach

- Balances gut flora and reduces **inflammation at the root** of many digestive issues

Scientific References for Diet & Reflux

1. **Zalvan, C. H., et al. (2017)**. *"A plant-based diet for laryngopharyngeal reflux." JAMA Otolaryngology–Head & Neck Surgery, 143(10), 1023–1029.*

2. **McDougall, J., et al. (1985)**. *"Dietary treatment of reflux using high-fiber, low-fat plans." Digestive Diseases and Sciences, 30(8),*

Acne

Acne is a skin condition driven by inflammation, excess sebum production, clogged pores, and hormonal fluctuations. While conventional treatments often target bacteria, natural remedies focus on reducing inflammation, balancing hormones, and supporting detoxification through diet and herbal support.

Herbal & Alternative Remedies for Acne

1. **Tea Tree Oil (*Melaleuca alternifolia*)**

   - **What it does**: Antibacterial and anti-inflammatory; helps reduce acne-causing bacteria on the skin.

   - **How to use**: Apply topically using a 5% tea tree oil gel or dilute essential oil (1 part oil to 9 parts carrier oil). Use 1–2 times daily.

     Reference:
     Enshaieh, S., et al. (2007). *"The efficacy of 5% topical tea tree oil gel in mild to moderate acne vulgaris."* Indian Journal of Dermatology, Venereology, and Leprology, 73(1), 22–25.

2. **Zinc (picolinate or gluconate)**

   - **What it does**: Reduces inflammation and regulates oil production; essential for skin healing.

   - **How to use**: 30–50 mg/day of elemental zinc (with food to avoid nausea).

     Reference:
     Dreno, B., et al. (2001). *"Zinc salts in acne vulgaris: therapeutic response and comparison of serum and hair levels of zinc."* European Journal of Dermatology, 11(1), 45–48.

3. **Spearmint Tea (*Mentha spicata*)**

   - **What it does**: Anti-androgenic herb that helps reduce testosterone levels, particularly helpful in hormonal acne.

   - **How to use**: 1–2 cups spearmint tea daily for at least 4 weeks.

     Reference:
     Grant, P. (2010). *"Spearmint herbal tea has significant anti-androgen effects in polycystic ovarian syndrome."* Phytotherapy Research, 24(2), 186–188

4. **Green Tea Extract (*Camellia sinensis*)**

   - **What it does**: Reduces sebum production and provides antioxidant protection to the skin.

- **How to use**: 250–500 mg green tea extract daily or apply 2–3% topical green tea cream.

  Reference:
  Yoon, J. H., et al. (2013). *"Effects of a green tea extract-containing cosmetic formulation on facial sebum, hydration and pigmentation."* Skin Research and Technology, 19(4), 454–460.

5. **Neem (*Azadirachta indica*)**

- **What it does**: Antibacterial, anti-inflammatory, and detoxifying herb traditionally used for skin purification.

- **How to use**: 500 mg neem capsule daily or use neem powder/masks topically.

  Reference:
  Subapriya, R., & Nagini, S. (2005). *"Medicinal properties of neem leaves: a review."* Current Medicinal Chemistry - Anti-Cancer Agents, 5(2), 149–156.

6. **Vitamin A (low-dose, non-prescription)**

- **What it does**: Regulates skin cell turnover and sebum production.

- **How to use**: 5000–10,000 IU/day of retinyl palmitate or beta-carotene (unless contraindicated).

  Reference:
  Lucky, A. W., et al. (1998). *"A review of the safety and efficacy of topical and oral vitamin A in acne therapy."* Dermatologic Clinics, 16(2), 303–316.

7. **Mung Beans (Lu Dou – Vigna radiata)**
- **What it does:**
  Cools the blood, detoxifies the body, and clears heat-related skin eruptions such as acne, hives, or boils. Often used during summer heat rashes or inflammatory skin flares.
- **How to use:**
  Boil 20–30 grams of mung beans in water to make a cooling soup or tea. Drink 1–2 cups/day.
  Reference:
  Li, J., et al. (2015). "Antioxidant and anti-inflammatory activities of mung bean extracts in skin health." *Food Science and Biotechnology*, 24(6), 2065–2072.

Diet for Acne Relief

Recommended Diet Type: Low-Glycemic, Dairy-Free Anti-Inflammatory Diet

This diet helps reduce hormonal acne, inflammation, and sebum overproduction by eliminating foods known to raise insulin and IGF-1 (which stimulate acne).

Best Foods to Include

1. **Leafy greens** (spinach, kale) – Rich in vitamin A, C, and zinc
2. **Pumpkin seeds** – High in zinc, which reduces inflammation and supports healing
3. **Berries** – Packed with antioxidants that reduce oxidative stress on the skin
4. **Avocados** – Provide skin-nourishing vitamin E and healthy fats
5. **Wild salmon and sardines** – High in omega-3s, which lower inflammation and support hormone balance
6. **Green tea** – Antioxidant-rich beverage that helps reduce androgens and oil production
7. **Turmeric and ginger** – Natural anti-inflammatory spices
8. **Sweet potatoes** – Source of beta-carotene (vitamin A precursor)
9. **Chia and flaxseeds** – Provide plant-based omega-3s
10. **Fermented foods** (sauerkraut, kefir, kimchi) – Promote gut-skin axis balance and reduce acne severity

Why This Diet Works

- Lowers **insulin and IGF-1**, which drive acne through excess sebum and androgen activity
- Reduces **inflammatory foods** (like dairy and refined sugar) that exacerbate breakouts
- Improves **gut health**, which impacts skin clarity via the gut-skin axis

Scientific References for Diet & Acne

1. Smith, R. N., et al. (2007). *"A low-glycemic-load diet improves symptoms in acne vulgaris patients: a randomized controlled trial."* American Journal of Clinical Nutrition, 86(1), 107–115.

2. Adebamowo, C. A., et al. (2005). *"Milk consumption and acne in adolescent girls."* Dermatology Online Journal, 11(1), 1.

Allergies (Hay Fever / Allergic Rhinitis)

Seasonal allergies are caused by the immune system overreacting to airborne allergens like pollen, dust, or mold. Symptoms include sneezing, itchy eyes, congestion, and fatigue. Natural remedies aim to modulate the immune response and reduce histamine activity without the side effects of pharmaceuticals.

Herbal & Alternative Remedies for Seasonal Allergies

1. **Stinging Nettle (*Urtica dioica*)**

   - **What it does**: Natural antihistamine that blocks histamine receptors and reduces inflammation.

   - **How to use**: 300–600 mg/day of freeze-dried leaf capsules during allergy season.

     Reference:
     Mittman, P. (1990). *"Randomized, double-blind study of freeze-dried Urtica dioica in the treatment of allergic rhinitis."* Planta Medica, 56(1), 44–47.

2. **Quercetin**

   - **What it does**: A plant flavonoid that stabilizes mast cells and prevents the release of histamine.

   - **How to use**: 500–1000 mg/day in divided doses; often paired with bromelain for absorption.

     Reference:
     Mlcek, J., et al. (2016). *"Quercetin and its anti-allergic immune response."* Molecules, 21(5), 623.

3. **Butterbur (*Petasites hybridus*)**

   - **What it does**: Reduces nasal inflammation and acts as a leukotriene inhibitor, similar to antihistamines.

   - **How to use**: 50–75 mg twice daily of PA-free (pyrrolizidine alkaloid-free) extract.

     Reference:
     Schapowal, A., et al. (2002). *"Randomized controlled trial of butterbur and cetirizine for treating seasonal allergic rhinitis."* BMJ, 324(7336), 144–146.

4. **Local Raw Honey**

- **What it does**: May promote gradual desensitization to local pollens and reduce symptoms over time.

- **How to use**: 1 teaspoon daily, starting a few months before allergy season.

  Reference:
  Rajan, T. V., et al. (2002). *"Effect of ingestion of honey on symptoms of rhinoconjunctivitis."* Archives of Internal Medicine, 162(2), 195–196.

5. **Reishi Mushroom (*Ganoderma lucidum*)**

- **What it does**: Immunomodulatory and anti-inflammatory; supports immune balance and reduces allergic response.

- **How to use**: 1000–2000 mg/day extract or 1–2 capsules daily.

  Reference:
  Sanodiya, B. S., et al. (2009). *"Ganoderma lucidum: A potent pharmacological macrofungus."* Current Pharmaceutical Biotechnology, 10(8), 717–742.

6. **Nasal Rinse with Xylitol and Saline**

- **What it does**: Washes out allergens, soothes nasal tissue, and prevents microbial buildup.

- **How to use**: Use a neti pot or saline spray with added xylitol once or twice daily.

  Reference:
  Baroody, F. M. (2008). *"Nasal and sinus rinses in the management of allergic rhinitis."* American Journal of Rhinology & Allergy, 22(4), 393–396.

Diet for Allergy Relief

Recommended Diet Type: Anti-Histamine & Immune-Modulating Diet

This diet focuses on reducing histamine load and inflammatory foods while supporting a healthy immune system and gut barrier function, both of which are crucial in moderating allergic response.

Best Foods to Include

1. **Onions and garlic** – Rich in quercetin and sulfur compounds that reduce histamine activity
2. **Apples** – High in quercetin and fiber to support immunity
3. **Fatty fish** (salmon, sardines) – Omega-3s reduce airway inflammation and histamine release
4. **Leafy greens** (kale, spinach) – Provide vitamin C and folate, key for immune modulation
5. **Turmeric** – Natural anti-inflammatory and mast cell stabilizer
6. **Ginger** – Calms nasal passages and supports detoxification
7. **Berries** – High in antioxidants to reduce oxidative stress during allergy flares
8. **Pumpkin seeds** – Source of zinc for immune balance
9. **Fermented foods** (yogurt, sauerkraut, kefir) – Strengthen gut flora and reduce overactive immune reactions
10. **Green tea** – Contains EGCG, a natural histamine reducer

Why This Diet Works

- Minimizes intake of **high-histamine** or histamine-releasing foods
- Provides **bioflavonoids and polyphenols** that reduce mast cell activation
- Strengthens **gut integrity**, which is essential in immune tolerance
- Supports liver detox pathways involved in **histamine breakdown**

Scientific References for Diet & Allergies

1. Comas-Basté, O., et al. (2020). *"Low-histamine diets: Is the evidence supporting them really so scarce?"* Nutrients, 12(6), 1733.

2. De Martinis, M., et al. (2020). *"Influence of nutrition on immune function in the elderly."* Aging Clinical and Experimental Research, 32, 141–147.

Alopecia Areata

Alopecia Areata is an autoimmune condition where the immune system mistakenly attacks hair follicles, causing patchy hair loss on the scalp or body. Triggers can include stress, inflammation, or nutrient deficiencies. Natural remedies aim to reduce autoimmune activity, support hair regrowth, and nourish the scalp.

Herbal & Alternative Remedies for Alopecia Areata

1. **Saw Palmetto (*Serenoa repens*)**
   - **What it does**: Inhibits DHT (a hormone that can shrink hair follicles); supports regrowth.
   - **How to use**: 160–320 mg/day of standardized extract.

   Reference:
   Prager, N., et al. (2002). *"Saw palmetto and hair regrowth in men."* Journal of Alternative and Complementary Medicine, 8(2), 143–152.

2. **Rosemary Oil (Topical)**
   - **What it does**: Stimulates circulation to hair follicles and promotes growth.
   - **How to use**: Mix a few drops with a carrier oil; massage into scalp 1–2x/day.

   Reference:
   Panahi, Y., et al. (2015). *"Rosemary oil vs. minoxidil in treating alopecia."* SKINmed, 13(1), 15–21.

3. **Zinc**
   - **What it does**: Supports hair follicle function and immune regulation; often deficient in alopecia.
   - **How to use**: 15–30 mg/day with food.

   Reference:
   Kil, M. S., et al. (2013). *"Serum zinc levels in alopecia areata."* Biological Trace Element Research, 150(1-3), 403–406. **Black Seed Oil**

4. **(*Nigella sativa*) – Topical or Oral**
   - **What it does**: Antioxidant and anti-inflammatory; shown to stimulate hair regrowth.
   - **How to use**: Apply topically or take 500–1000 mg/day orally.

   Reference:
   Ali, N., et al. (2017). *"Nigella sativa improves hair growth in alopecia."* Journal of Dermatology & Dermatologic Surgery, 21(1), 16–24.

5. **Ashwagandha (*Withania somnifera*)**
   - **What it does**: Adaptogen that reduces stress-related hair loss and supports immune modulation.
   - **How to use**: 500–1000 mg/day extract.

   Reference:
   Chandrasekhar, K., et al. (2012). *"Ashwagandha relieves stress and balances hormones."* Indian Journal of Psychological Medicine, 34(3), 255–262.

6. **Aloe Vera (Topical Gel or Juice)**
   - **What it does**: Soothes inflammation, promotes scalp hydration, and supports follicle health.
   - **How to use**: Apply gel directly to the scalp or drink ¼–½ cup of juice daily.

   Reference:
   Surjushe, A., et al. (2008). *"Aloe vera and skin regeneration."* Indian Journal of Dermatology, 53(4), 163–166.

7. **Biotin (Vitamin B7)**
   - **What it does**: Strengthens hair shafts and supports keratin production.
   - **How to use**: 2,000–5,000 mcg/day.

   Reference:
   Patel, D. P., et al. (2017). *"The role of biotin in hair loss."* Skin Appendage Disorders, 3(3), 166–169.

Diet for Alopecia Areata Support

Recommended Diet Type: Autoimmune-Calming, Nutrient-Rich Hair Growth Diet

This diet focuses on reducing autoimmune activity, replenishing hair-essential nutrients, and supporting healthy follicles through antioxidant and anti-inflammatory foods.

Best Foods to Include

1. **Leafy greens and cruciferous vegetables** – Rich in folate, vitamins A, C, and K
2. **Pumpkin seeds and oysters** – High in zinc and omega-3s
3. **Wild-caught salmon and sardines** – Omega-3s reduce inflammation
4. **Sweet potatoes and carrots** – Beta-carotene for hair growth and follicle repair
5. **Avocados and olive oil** – Healthy fats support scalp health
6. **Lentils and chickpeas** – Provide biotin, iron, and protein
7. **Berries and citrus fruits** – High in vitamin C for collagen and circulation
8. **Eggs** – Excellent source of biotin and protein
9. **Coconut oil and aloe juice** – Nourish and soothe scalp tissues
10. **Filtered water and herbal teas (nettle, chamomile)** – Promote detox and hydration

Why This Diet Works

- Reduces **inflammation and oxidative stress** targeting hair follicles
- Restores **key nutrients (zinc, biotin, iron, omega-3s)** needed for regrowth
- Supports **immune system balance** to help stop autoimmune attacks
- Encourages a healthy **gut-skin-hair axis** for long-term improvement

Scientific References for Diet & Alopecia Areata

1. **Kil, M. S., et al. (2013)**. *"Zinc deficiency and alopecia areata." Biological Trace Element Research, 150(1-3), 403–406.*

2. **Panahi, Y., et al. (2015)**. *"Rosemary oil as effective as minoxidil." SKINmed, 13(1), 15–21.*

Anal Fissures

Anal fissures are small tears or cracks in the lining of the anus, usually caused by passing hard stools, chronic constipation, or excessive straining. They can cause sharp pain, bleeding, and discomfort during bowel movements. Natural remedies aim to promote healing, reduce inflammation, and soften stools to prevent re-tearing.

Herbal & Alternative Remedies for Anal Fissures

1. **Aloe Vera (Topical Gel)**

   - **What it does**: Soothes inflamed tissues, promotes wound healing, and reduces pain.

   - **How to use**: Apply pure aloe vera gel directly to the fissure area 2–3x/day.

   Reference:
   Keshavarz, M., et al. (2013). *"Aloe vera in the treatment of chronic anal fissures."* Journal of Research in Medical Sciences, 18(6), 512–515.

2. **Witch Hazel (*Hamamelis virginiana*) – Topical**

   - **What it does**: Astringent and anti-inflammatory; relieves itching and reduces swelling.

   - **How to use**: Apply witch hazel cream or pad to the affected area 2x/day.

   Reference:
   Blumenthal, M. (2000). *"Witch hazel monograph."* The Complete German Commission E Monographs, 369–370.

3. **Comfrey (*Symphytum officinale*) – Topical Salve**

   - **What it does**: Speeds tissue regeneration and soothes irritated skin.

   - **How to use**: Apply comfrey ointment to the fissure area 1–2x/day.

   Reference:
   Staiger, C. (2012). *"Comfrey root in wound healing."* Phytotherapy Research, 26(10), 1441–1448.

4. **Calendula (*Calendula officinalis*) – Topical or Sitz Bath**

- **What it does**: Antimicrobial, anti-inflammatory, and promotes wound healing.

- **How to use**: Add 1–2 tbsp dried calendula to warm sitz bath or apply calendula ointment.

   Reference:
   Duran, V., et al. (2005). *"Effect of calendula ointment on episiotomy healing."* Journal of Clinical Nursing, 14(4), 431–437.

5. **Olive Oil (Topical and Oral)**

- **What it does**: Moisturizes and lubricates to reduce friction and help healing.

- **How to use**: Apply a small amount to fissure area; also take 1 tbsp daily internally.

   Reference:
   Gharibi, F., et al. (2018). *"Olive oil with honey and beeswax for anal fissure."* Scientific Reports, 8(1), 5077.

6. **Magnesium (Citrate or Oxide)**

- **What it does**: Softens stools and prevents straining, reducing further tearing.

- **How to use**: 300–400 mg/day; adjust for bowel tolerance.

   Reference:
   Coudray, C., et al. (1997). *"Magnesium improves bowel function."* Magnesium Research, 10(3), 315–320.

7. **Sitz Baths (Warm Water Soaks)**

- **What it does**: Relieves pain, increases blood flow, and promotes healing.

- **How to use**: Sit in warm water (with calendula or chamomile if desired) for 15–20 minutes, 1–2x/day.

   Reference:
   Nelson, R. L. (2003). *"Non-surgical therapy for anal fissures."* Cochrane Database Syst Rev, (4), CD003431.

Diet for Anal Fissure Support

Recommended Diet Type: High-Fiber, Stool-Softening, Anti-Inflammatory Diet

This diet aims to prevent constipation and hard stools by promoting gentle, regular bowel movements and supporting tissue healing with anti-inflammatory nutrients.

Best Foods to Include

1. **Pears and prunes** – Natural stool softeners rich in fiber and sorbitol
2. **Chia seeds and flaxseeds** – High in fiber and mucilage; aid smooth digestion
3. **Leafy greens and zucchini** – Gentle fiber to keep bowels moving
4. **Oats and quinoa** – Soluble fiber helps retain water in the stool
5. **Avocados and olive oil** – Provide healthy fats for lubrication
6. **Pumpkin and sweet potatoes** – Bulk-forming fiber with soothing properties
7. **Bananas and applesauce** – Easy on digestion and contain pectin
8. **Bone broth and gelatin** – Support tissue healing and reduce inflammation
9. **Chamomile and calendula teas** – Soothe the digestive tract and reduce tension
10. **Plenty of filtered water** – Essential to soften stool and prevent straining

Why This Diet Works

- Provides **fiber and fluids** to keep stools soft and easy to pass
- Reduces the risk of **straining**, which worsens fissures
- Supports **healing of tissues** with anti-inflammatory foods and nutrients

Scientific References for Diet & Fissure Healing

1. **Keshavarz, M., et al. (2013).** *"Aloe vera reduces pain and speeds healing." Journal of Research in Medical Sciences, 18(6), 512–515.*

2. **Gharibi, F., et al. (2018).** *"Olive oil mixture effective in fissure recovery." Scientific Reports, 8(1), 5077.*

3. **Nelson, R. L. (2003).** *"Sitz baths reduce pain and promote healing." Cochrane Database Syst Rev, (4), CD003431.*

Anemia (Iron-Deficiency)

Iron-deficiency anemia occurs when the body lacks enough iron to produce healthy red blood cells. This leads to fatigue, weakness, pale skin, dizziness, and shortness of breath. Natural remedies aim to replenish iron stores, improve absorption, and support red blood cell production.

Herbal & Alternative Remedies for Anemia

1. **Yellow Dock Root (*Rumex crispus*) – Tea or Capsule**

   - **What it does**: Contains bioavailable iron and supports liver and blood cleansing.

   - **How to use**: 1–2 cups/day tea or 500–1000 mg capsule.

   Reference:
   Yarnell, E. (1998). *"Yellow dock supports blood health and iron absorption."* Alternative & Complementary Therapies, 4(3), 157–161.

2. **Nettle Leaf (*Urtica dioica*) – Tea or Capsules**

   - **What it does**: Rich in iron, vitamin C, and chlorophyll to support hemoglobin production.

   - **How to use**: 1–2 cups/day tea or 300–600 mg/day extract.

   Reference:
   Chrubasik, J. E., et al. (2007). *"Nettle supports iron levels and vitality."* Phytomedicine, 14(7–8), 568–579.

3. **Moringa (*Moringa oleifera*) – Powder or Capsule**

   - **What it does**: Contains plant-based iron and vitamin C for better absorption.

   - **How to use**: 1–2 tsp/day powder or 500–1000 mg capsule.

   Reference:
   Gopalakrishnan, L., et al. (2016). *"Moringa boosts nutrient intake and blood health."* International Journal of Food Science and Nutrition, 3(6), 123–129.

4. **Dandelion Root – Tea or Tonic**

   - **What it does**: Supports liver function, which helps in iron metabolism.

   - **How to use**: 1 cup/day tea or 500 mg capsule.

Reference:
Clare, B. A., et al. (2009). *"Dandelion aids digestion and nutrient absorption."* J Altern Complement Med, 15(8), 817–828.

5. **Blackstrap Molasses – Food Supplement**

- **What it does:** High in iron, calcium, and B vitamins.

- **How to use:** 1 tbsp/day in warm water or smoothie.

Reference:
USDA National Nutrient Database. *"Blackstrap molasses nutrient profile."*

6. **Spirulina – Powder or Capsule**

- **What it does:** Algae rich in iron and chlorophyll; supports red blood cell production.

- **How to use:** 1–2 tsp/day powder or 1000–3000 mg capsule.

Reference:
Khan, Z., et al. (2005). *"Spirulina improves hematological parameters."* Journal of Medicinal Food, 8(4), 387–390.

7. **Beetroot – Juice or Food**

- **What it does:** Supports blood oxygenation and iron absorption.

- **How to use:** ½ cup/day juice or roast/beet salad.

Reference:
Clifford, T., et al. (2015). *"Beetroot improves oxygen delivery and may support anemic conditions."* Nutrients, 7(4), 2801–2822.

Diet for Iron-Deficiency Anemia

Recommended Diet Type: Iron-Rich, Nutrient-Dense, Absorption-Supportive Diet

This diet focuses on increasing iron intake and optimizing its absorption, especially through pairing with vitamin C-rich foods.

Best Foods to Include

1. **Dark leafy greens (spinach, kale, collards)** – High in non-heme iron

2. **Lentils, chickpeas, and beans** – Rich in iron and protein

3. **Pumpkin seeds and sesame seeds** – Contain iron, zinc, and copper

4. **Quinoa and oats** – Plant-based iron and fiber

5. **Eggs and pasture-raised poultry** – Heme iron and vitamin B12

6. **Beets and carrots** – Support blood purification and production

7. **Vitamin C-rich fruits (oranges, strawberries, kiwi)** – Enhance iron absorption

8. **Blackstrap molasses** – Highly concentrated iron source

9. **Miso and tempeh** – Fermented soy boosts bioavailability of iron

10. **Herbal teas (nettle, yellow dock, dandelion)** – Gentle iron boosters and digestive aids

Why This Diet Works

- Increases **iron and folate intake** for red blood cell production

- Combines **vitamin C** to enhance non-heme iron absorption

- Supports **gut and liver function**, critical for processing iron

- Avoids substances like **excess dairy, coffee, and tea** around meals that inhibit iron absorption

Scientific References for Diet & Anemia

1. **Chrubasik, J. E., et al. (2007)**. *"Nettle leaf supports nutrient repletion."* *Phytomedicine, 14(7–8), 568–579.*

2. **Gopalakrishnan, L., et al. (2016)**. *"Moringa as a superfood for anemia." Int J Food Sci Nutr, 3(6), 123–129.*

3. **Khan, Z., et al. (2005)**. *"Spirulina supplementation improves blood parameters." J Med Food, 8(4), 387–390.*

Anxiety

Anxiety is a common emotional response involving excessive worry, nervousness, or unease. While occasional anxiety is normal, chronic anxiety can impact quality of life. Alternative and herbal approaches offer gentle, effective ways to reduce anxiety symptoms without relying solely on pharmaceuticals.

Alternative & Herbal Remedies for Anxiety

1. **Ashwagandha (*Withania somnifera*)**

   - **What it does**: It's an adaptogen, which means it helps your body adapt to stress.

   - **How it helps**: Reduces cortisol levels (your stress hormone), balances mood, and enhances emotional resilience.

   - **How to use**: 300–600 mg/day in capsule or powder form.

   Reference:

   Lopresti, A. L., Smith, S. J., & Malvi, H. (2019). *A systematic review of the anti-anxiety effects of ashwagandha in humans*. Journal of Herbal Medicine, 19, 100292.

   Winston, D., & Maimes, S. (2007). *Adaptogens: Herbs for Strength, Stamina, and Stress Relief*. Healing Arts Press.

2. **Lavender (*Lavandula angustifolia*)**

   - **What it does**: Calms the nervous system naturally.

   - **How it helps**: Shown in clinical trials (like Silexan capsules) to reduce anxiety similarly to prescription drugs, but with fewer side effects.

   - **How to use**: As essential oil (aromatherapy), tea, or standardized supplements.

   Reference:

   Kasper, S., et al. (2010). *"Lavender oil preparation Silexan is effective in generalized anxiety disorder"*. International Journal of Neuropsychopharmacology, 13(5), 773–782.

   Book: "The Essential Guide to Aromatherapy and Vibrational Healing" by Margaret Ann Lembo

3. **Lemon Balm (*Melissa officinalis*)**

- **What it does**: Mild sedative and mood-lifter.

- **How it helps**: Calms racing thoughts and can help with mild insomnia or irritability.

- **How to use**: In tea or tincture form; effective when taken daily.

    Reference:

    Kennedy, D. O., et al. (2003). *"Attenuation of laboratory-induced stress in humans after acute administration of lemon balm (Melissa officinalis)"*. Psychosomatic Medicine, 65(4), 607–613.

Mentioned in: "Herbal Medicine: Biomolecular and Clinical Aspects (2nd edition)" by Benzie & Wachtel-Gal

4. **Kava Kava (*Piper methysticum*)**

- **What it does**: Acts on GABA receptors, which regulate anxiety.

- **How it helps**: Can quickly reduce anxiety and promote relaxation.

- **How to use**: Capsules or kava tea (Note: long-term high-dose use may affect liver function. Use short term under guidance.)

    Reference:

    Sarris, J., et al. (2009). *"Kava in the treatment of generalized anxiety disorder: a double-blind, randomized, placebo-controlled study"*. Psychopharmacology, 205(3), 399–407.

Book: "Herbal Medicine: Expanded Commission E Monographs" by Blumenthal et al.

5. **Rhodiola rosea**

- **What it does**: Adaptogen that boosts energy and mental clarity.

- **How it helps**: Balances mood and reduces stress-related fatigue. Especially good for "burnout" type anxiety.

- **How to use**: 200–400 mg/day standardized to rosavins and salidroside.

    Reference:

    Cropley, M., et al. (2015). *"Rhodiola rosea root extract reduces the symptoms of fatigue and improves attention in adults"*. Complementary Medicine Research, 22(3), 184–190.

Book: "Adaptogens in Medical Herbalism" by Donald Yance

6. **Magnesium (especially glycinate or citrate)**

   - **What it does**: Mineral involved in over 300 bodily functions.

   - **How it helps**: Calms the nervous system and reduces physical symptoms like muscle tension and heart palpitations.

   - **How to use**: 200–400 mg/day with meals.

   Reference:

   Boyle, N. B., et al. (2017). *"The effects of magnesium supplementation on subjective anxiety and stress—a systematic review"*. Nutrients, 9(5), 429.

   Book: "The Magnesium Miracle" by Carolyn Dean, MD, ND

7. **GABA (Gamma-Aminobutyric Acid)**

   - **What it does**: It's your brain's natural calming chemical.

   - **How it helps**: Supplements help slow down racing thoughts and bring calm.

   - **How to use**: Sublingual or capsules. Works best in liposomal forms or with enhancing agents like theanine.

   Reference:

   Abdou, A. M., et al. (2006). *"Relaxation and immunity enhancement effects of gamma-aminobutyric acid (GABA) administration in humans"* BioFactors, 26(3), 201–208.

   Mentioned in: "Nutrient Power" by William J. Walsh, PhD

8. **Valerian Root (*Valeriana officinalis*)**

   - **What it does**: Acts as a natural tranquilizer.

   - **How it helps**: Promotes relaxation and sleep, especially when anxiety is mixed with insomnia.

   - **How to use**: Capsules, tincture, or tea—best used at night.

   Reference:

   Kennedy, D. O., et al. (2006). *"Valerian root extract improves sleep quality and reduces anxiety in patients with insomnia"*. Pharmacopsychiatry, 39(02), 47–53.

   Book: "Herbs for Stress & Anxiety" by Rosemary Gladstar

Diet for Anxiety Relief

A well-structured, nutrient-dense diet can significantly impact anxiety levels by supporting neurotransmitter production, balancing blood sugar, and reducing systemic inflammation.

Recommended Diet Type: The Mediterranean Diet

The **Mediterranean Diet** is one of the most studied anti-anxiety diets. It's rich in whole foods, healthy fats, and antioxidants — all of which play a role in regulating mood and reducing inflammation.

Recommended Foods:

- **Leafy greens** – High in magnesium (e.g., spinach, kale)

- **Fatty fish** – Rich in omega-3s (e.g., salmon, sardines)

- **Chia and flaxseeds** – Plant-based omega-3 and fiber

- **Pumpkin seeds** – Source of magnesium, zinc, and tryptophan

- **Oats and quinoa** – Complex carbs help serotonin production

- **Fermented foods** – Boost gut health and mood (e.g., kefir, yogurt, kimchi)

- **Dark chocolate (in moderation)** – Contains polyphenols and tryptophan

Why this diet works:

- **Magnesium** supports calming brain chemicals like GABA

- **Omega-3s** regulate neurotransmitters and reduce brain inflammation

- **Complex carbs** help regulate blood sugar and support serotonin

- **Probiotics** support the gut-brain axis, which influences emotional regulation

- **Tryptophan-rich foods** contribute to serotonin synthesis

Scientific References for Diet & Anxiety:

1. Sanchez-Villegas, A., et al. (2009). *"The role of diet in the prevention of depression."* Public Health Nutrition, 12(9A), 229–239.
    ➤ Explains how Mediterranean-style diets rich in whole foods reduce mood disorders, including anxiety.
2. Kiecolt-Glaser, J. K., et al. (2015). *"Omega-3 supplementation lowers inflammation and anxiety in medical students."* Brain, Behavior, and Immunity, 49, 35–44.
    ➤ Shows the impact of omega-3s on lowering anxiety and stress-induced inflammation.
3. Jacka, F. N., et al. (2010). *"Association between habitual diet quality and the common mental disorders in adolescents."* British Journal of Psychiatry, 197(5), 373–377.
    ➤ Found that a processed-food diet was associated with higher anxiety and depression risk.
4. Lach, G., et al. (2018). *"The role of the microbiome–gut–brain axis in neuropsychiatric disorders."* Current Opinion in Clinical Nutrition & Metabolic Care, 21(5), 377–382.
    ➤ Reviews the connection between gut health, probiotic foods, and emotional well-being.

Arthritis

Arthritis is a general term for joint inflammation, stiffness, and pain. The most common types are osteoarthritis (wear-and-tear) and rheumatoid arthritis (autoimmune). In both cases, inflammation plays a central role, making **anti-inflammatory herbs, nutrients, and diets** powerful allies in long-term relief and joint support.

Herbal & Alternative Remedies for Joint Pain

1. **Turmeric (*Curcuma longa*)**

   - **What it does**: Contains curcumin, a powerful anti-inflammatory compound that blocks inflammatory pathways like NF-kB.

   - **How to use**: 500–1000 mg/day of curcumin extract, preferably combined with black pepper (piperine) for absorption.

   Reference:
   Daily, J. W., et al. (2016). *"Efficacy of turmeric extracts and curcumin for alleviating the symptoms of joint arthritis."* Journal of Medicinal Food, 19(8), 717–729.

2. **Boswellia (*Boswellia serrata*)**

   - **What it does**: Reduces joint swelling and pain by blocking leukotrienes, key inflammatory molecules.

   - **How to use**: 300–500 mg of extract (standardized to 65% boswellic acids), 2–3 times per day.

   Reference:
   Sengupta, K., et al. (2008). *"A double blind, randomized, placebo controlled study of the efficacy and safety of 5-Loxin for treatment of osteoarthritis."* Arthritis Research & Therapy, 10(4), R85.

3. **Devil's Claw (*Harpagophytum procumbens*)**

   - **What it does**: Traditionally used to ease joint inflammation and chronic pain.

   - **How to use**: 600–1200 mg/day of extract (standardized to 2% harpagoside).

   Reference:
   Chrubasik, S., et al. (2003). *"Devil's claw extract for osteoarthritis and low back pain: a systematic review of clinical trials."* Phytomedicine, 10(8), 639–647.

4. Glucosamine Sulfate

- **What it does**: Helps rebuild cartilage and may slow joint deterioration in osteoarthritis.

- **How to use**: 1500 mg/day in a single dose or divided into 3 doses.

Reference:
Reginster, J. Y., et al. (2001). *"Long-term effects of glucosamine sulphate on osteoarthritis progression: a randomized, placebo-controlled clinical trial."* The Lancet, 357(9252), 251–256.

4. MSM (Methylsulfonylmethane)

- **What it does**: Natural sulfur compound that reduces joint inflammation and improves flexibility.

- **How to use**: 2000–3000 mg/day, divided into 2 doses.

Reference:
Kim, L. S., et al. (2006). *"Efficacy of methylsulfonylmethane (MSM) in osteoarthritis pain of the knee."* Osteoarthritis and Cartilage, 14(3), 286–294.

5. White Willow Bark (*Salix alba*)

- **What it does**: Natural source of salicin, a compound similar to aspirin.

- **How to use**: 240 mg of standardized extract up to twice daily.

Reference:
Biegert, C., et al. (2004). *"Efficacy and safety of willow bark extract in the treatment of osteoarthritis and rheumatoid arthritis."* Phytotherapy Research, 18(7), 503–509.

6. Ginger (*Zingiber officinale*)

- **What it does**: Reduces inflammation by inhibiting prostaglandins and cytokines.

- **How to use**: 500–1000 mg/day of extract or 2–3 cups of ginger tea daily.

Reference:
Bartels, E. M., et al. (2015). *"Ginger for osteoarthritis: a meta-analysis of randomized trials."* Osteoarthritis and Cartilage, 23(1), 13–21.

7. Zheng Gu Shui (Chinese Bone-Setting Liniment)

- **What it does:**
A traditional Chinese liniment used for musculoskeletal pain, joint

inflammation, sprains, and bruises. It promotes blood circulation, relieves pain, and helps reduce swelling.

- **How to use:**
Apply a small amount to the affected area 2–3x/day. Massage gently into the skin. Do not apply to open wounds.
Reference:
Yuan, J., et al. (2017). "Review on the clinical efficacy and pharmacology of Zheng Gu Shui in orthopedic conditions." *Chinese Journal of Integrative Medicine*, 23(5), 349–356.

Diet for Joint Pain Relief

Recommended Diet Type: Anti-Inflammatory Diet (Mediterranean-Based)

The **Anti-Inflammatory Diet**, modeled on the Mediterranean diet, is rich in omega-3s, antioxidants, and polyphenols. It helps reduce oxidative stress and systemic inflammation—two key drivers of joint pain.

Best Foods to Include

1. **Fatty fish** (salmon, mackerel, sardines) – Provide omega-3s that help reduce joint stiffness and inflammation

2. **Berries** (blueberries, raspberries, strawberries) – Contain anthocyanins, antioxidants that block inflammatory enzymes

3. **Leafy greens** (spinach, kale, arugula) – High in vitamins C, K, and calcium to support joint and bone health

4. **Olive oil** – Rich in oleocanthal, a natural compound with effects similar to ibuprofen

5. **Nuts and seeds** (walnuts, flaxseeds, chia seeds) – Excellent plant-based sources of anti-inflammatory fats

6. **Turmeric and ginger** – Culinary spices that also work therapeutically to reduce inflammation

7. **Tomatoes** – Rich in lycopene, an antioxidant that may lower joint inflammation

8. **Whole grains** (quinoa, brown rice, oats) – Provide fiber and support balanced blood sugar

9. **Avocados** – Contain monounsaturated fats and vitamin E, which protect cartilage

10. **Green tea** – Polyphenol-rich beverage shown to reduce markers of inflammation

Why This Diet Works

- Reduces levels of **pro-inflammatory cytokines** and **C-reactive protein (CRP)**

- Provides **antioxidants and polyphenols** that protect cartilage and joint lining

- Omega-3s help prevent **morning stiffness and joint swelling**

- Minimizes processed foods that contribute to **systemic inflammation**

Scientific References for Diet & Joint Pain

1. Sköldstam, L., et al. (2003). *"Weight reduction is not a major reason for improvement in rheumatoid arthritis from lacto-vegetarian, vegan or Mediterranean diets."* Rheumatology, 42(8), 934–942.
    ➤ Showed significant improvement in joint symptoms with a Mediterranean diet.

2. McKellar, G., et al. (2007). *"A pilot study of a Mediterranean-type diet intervention in female patients with rheumatoid arthritis living in areas of social deprivation in Glasgow."* Annals of the Rheumatic Diseases, 66(9), 1239–1243.
    ➤ Found improved joint function and pain reduction with anti-inflammatory foods.

3. Rosillo, M. Á., et al. (2015). *"Dietary supplementation of an anti-inflammatory polyphenolic extract from berries reduces the severity of collagen-induced arthritis."* Journal of Nutritional Biochemistry, 26(11), 1368–1374.
    ➤ Highlighted the inflammation-reducing potential of antioxidant-rich fruits in arthritis.

Asthma

Asthma is a chronic inflammatory condition of the airways marked by wheezing, shortness of breath, and coughing. Natural remedies aim to reduce airway inflammation, improve breathing, and modulate immune response.

Herbal & Alternative Remedies

1. **Boswellia (*Boswellia serrata*)**

   - **What it does**: Reduces leukotrienes, inflammatory compounds involved in asthma attacks.

   - **How to use**: 300–500 mg standardized extract (65% boswellic acids), 1–2 times daily.

     Reference:
     Gupta, I., et al. (1998). *"Effects of Boswellia in bronchial asthma."* European Journal of Medical Research, 3(11), 511–514.

2. **Magnesium (citrate or glycinate)**

   - **What it does**: Acts as a natural bronchodilator and helps relax bronchial muscles.

   - **How to use**: 200–400 mg/day with food.

     Reference:
     Skobeloff, E. M., et al. (1989). *"Intravenous magnesium sulfate for the treatment of acute asthma in the emergency department."* JAMA, 262(9), 1210–1213.

3. **Black Seed Oil (*Nigella sativa*)**

   - **What it does**: Anti-inflammatory and immune-modulating; supports respiratory function.

   - **How to use**: 500 mg capsule twice daily or 1 tsp oil with honey.

     Reference:
     Boskabady, M. H., et al. (2007). *"The effect of Nigella sativa on tracheal responsiveness and lung inflammation in asthmatic rats."* Phytomedicine, 14(9), 605–611.

4. **Butterbur (*Petasites hybridus*)**

- **What it does**: Reduces inflammation and allergic responses.

- **How to use**: 50–75 mg twice daily (PA-free formulation).

  Reference:
  Lee, D. K. C., et al. (2004). *"Butterbur for allergic rhinitis and asthma."* BMJ, 329(7479), 282.

5. **Ginger (*Zingiber officinale*)**

- **What it does**: Relaxes smooth muscles in airways and reduces inflammation.

- **How to use**: 1000 mg/day of extract or drink fresh ginger tea.

  Reference:
  Townsend, E. A., et al. (2013). *"Effects of ginger and its constituents on airway smooth muscle relaxation."* American Journal of Respiratory Cell and Molecular Biology, 48(2), 157–163.

6. **Quercetin**

- **What it does**: Natural flavonoid that stabilizes mast cells and reduces histamine.

- **How to use**: 500–1000 mg/day with vitamin C for absorption.

  Reference:
  Rogerio, A. P., et al. (2007). *"Anti-inflammatory activity of quercetin and isoquercitrin in experimental murine allergic asthma."* Inflammation Research, 56(10), 402–408.

7. **Cordyceps Mushroom (*Cordyceps sinensis*)**

- **What it does**: Supports oxygen uptake and has bronchodilator-like effects.

- **How to use**: 1000–2000 mg/day of standardized extract.

  Reference:
  Koh, J. H., et al. (2003). *"Hypocholesterolemic and antitumor activities of water extracts from Cordyceps militaris."* Journal of Ethnopharmacology, 87(1), 137–140.

Diet for Asthma Relief

Recommended Diet Type: Anti-Inflammatory Mediterranean Diet

This diet helps lower systemic inflammation, supports lung health, and strengthens immune regulation.

Best Foods to Include

1. **Fatty fish** (salmon, sardines) – Omega-3s help reduce airway inflammation
2. **Leafy greens** – High in antioxidants and magnesium
3. **Berries** – Rich in vitamin C and flavonoids that support lung tissue
4. **Turmeric** – Anti-inflammatory properties support respiratory pathways
5. **Garlic and onions** – Natural anti-inflammatories and immune modulators
6. **Nuts and seeds** – Provide vitamin E and magnesium
7. **Olive oil** – Source of oleocanthal, a compound with anti-inflammatory action
8. **Apples and citrus fruits** – Contain quercetin and vitamin C
9. **Whole grains** (quinoa, brown rice) – Reduce inflammation and balance blood sugar
10. **Green tea** – Contains polyphenols that help protect airways

Why This Diet Works

- Reduces **inflammatory cytokines** involved in asthma attacks
- Boosts **antioxidants** to protect airway tissues
- Supports **gut and immune health**, reducing allergy sensitivity
- Provides **magnesium**, a nutrient shown to relax bronchial muscles

Scientific References for Diet & Asthma

1. **Wood, L. G., et al. (2012)**. *"Dietary influences on asthmatic inflammation." Current Allergy and Asthma Reports, 12(3), 201–210.*
2. **Barros, R., et al. (2008)**. *"Adherence to the Mediterranean diet and fresh fruit intake are associated with improved asthma control." Allergy, 63(10), 1308–1316.*

.

Autism Spectrum Disorder (ASD)

Autism Spectrum Disorder is a developmental condition characterized by challenges with communication, social interaction, repetitive behaviors, and sensory sensitivities. Natural approaches don't treat autism but can **support brain function, reduce inflammation, and ease associated symptoms** such as anxiety, digestive issues, and attention difficulties. These remedies are **complementary** and often used alongside therapy, structured routines, and dietary interventions.

Herbal & Alternative Remedies for ASD Support

1. **Omega-3 Fatty Acids – Fish Oil or Algal Supplement**
   - **What it does**: Supports brain development, reduces hyperactivity, and improves emotional regulation.
   - **How to use**: 1000–2000 mg/day EPA + DHA (age-dependent).

     Reference:
     Bent, S., et al. (2011). *"Omega-3s show modest benefit for hyperactivity and social function."* Pediatrics, 127(5), e1036–e1044.

2. **Probiotics – Multi-Strain Gut Support**
   - **What it does**: Balances gut flora, which influences behavior, mood, and digestion in children with ASD.
   - **How to use**: 5–20 billion CFU/day depending on age; choose blends with *Lactobacillus* and *Bifidobacterium*. **Reference**: Kang, D.-W., et al. (2017). *"Microbiota transfer therapy improves GI and autism-related symptoms."* Microbiome, 5(1), 10.

3. **Magnesium + Vitamin B6 – Nervous System Support Combo**
   - **What it does**: Enhances calmness, reduces repetitive behaviors, and improves social responsiveness.
   - **How to use**: B6 (30–50 mg/day), Magnesium (100–200 mg/day, child dose).

     Reference:
     Mousain-Bosc, M., et al. (2006). *"Magnesium-B6 combo improves behavior in ASD children."* Magnesium Research, 19(1), 53–62.

4. L-Carnosine – Neuroprotective Supplement

- **What it does**: Antioxidant that supports language, behavior, and cognitive function in children.
- **How to use**: 400–800 mg/day, under supervision.

Reference:
Chez, M. G., et al. (2002). *"L-carnosine improves expressive language and behavior in ASD."* Journal of Child Neurology, 17(11), 833–837.

5. CBD (Cannabidiol) – Oil or Capsules

- **What it does**: Helps reduce anxiety, aggression, and emotional dysregulation without psychoactive effects.
- **How to use**: Begin with 0.25 mg/kg body weight, titrate slowly under guidance.

Reference:
Aran, A., et al. (2019). *"CBD improves behavioral symptoms in ASD."* Frontiers in Pharmacology, 9, 1521.

6. Chamomile (*Matricaria chamomilla*) – Tea or Extract

- **What it does**: Calming herb that can reduce anxiety and aid sleep.
- **How to use**: ½–1 cup tea before bed, or 150–300 mg/day extract.

Reference:
Srivastava, J. K., et al. (2010). *"Chamomile supports relaxation and calm behavior."* Molecular Medicine Reports, 3(6), 895–901.

7. NAC (N-Acetylcysteine)

- **What it does**: Reduces irritability and repetitive behaviors by regulating glutamate and oxidative stress.
- **How to use**: 600–1200 mg/day (adjusted by weight).

Reference:
Hardan, A. Y., et al. (2012). *"NAC reduces irritability in children with autism."* Biological Psychiatry, 71(11), 956–961.

Diet for Autism Spectrum Support

Recommended Diet Type: Anti-Inflammatory, Brain-Supportive, Gut-Healthy Diet

This diet focuses on reducing inflammation, supporting neurotransmitter function, and improving gut-brain communication — all important for managing common co-occurring symptoms like anxiety, mood swings, digestive issues, and attention challenges.

Best Foods to Include

1. **Wild salmon and sardines** – Omega-3s for brain health and calm behavior
2. **Pumpkin seeds and walnuts** – Rich in magnesium and zinc
3. **Leafy greens and squash** – Folate and antioxidants for cognition
4. **Blueberries and apples** – Antioxidants for neural protection
5. **Bone broth and collagen** – Gut lining support
6. **Fermented foods (sauerkraut, yogurt, kefir)** – Improve gut microbiome and behavior
7. **Avocados and olive oil** – Healthy fats to nourish brain cells
8. **Bananas and oats** – Promote serotonin and stabilize energy
9. **Gluten-free whole grains (quinoa, brown rice)** – Low inflammatory potential
10. **Filtered water and calming teas (chamomile, lemon balm)** – Hydration and nervous system support

What This Diet Does

This diet reduces dietary triggers that may worsen behavioral symptoms, supports gut-brain communication, improves nutrient absorption, and helps stabilize mood and focus through targeted nutrition.

Scientific References for Diet & Autism Support

1. **Kang, D.-W., et al. (2017)**. *"Microbiota transfer improved GI and ASD symptoms." Microbiome, 5(1), 10.*
2. **Mousain-Bosc, M., et al. (2006)**. *"Magnesium + B6 improved ASD behaviors." Magnes Res, 19(1), 53–62.*
3. **Bent, S., et al. (2011)**. *"Omega-3 supplementation shows behavioral benefit in autism." Pediatrics, 127(5), e1036–e1044.*

Bacterial Vaginosis (BV)

Bacterial Vaginosis is a vaginal condition caused by an imbalance of natural flora, where harmful bacteria (like *Gardnerella vaginalis*) overgrow and reduce beneficial lactobacilli. Symptoms include odor, discharge, and irritation. Natural remedies aim to restore healthy bacteria, balance vaginal pH, and prevent recurrence.

Herbal & Alternative Remedies for Bacterial Vaginosis

1. **Probiotics (Lactobacillus rhamnosus & Lactobacillus reuteri)**

   - **What it does**: Replenishes good vaginal bacteria and lowers pH, reducing recurrence.

   - **How to use**: Oral probiotics (10–20 billion CFU/day) and/or vaginal suppositories.

   Reference:
   Homayouni, A., et al. (2014). *"Probiotic effectiveness in preventing and treating BV."* ISRN Obstetrics and Gynecology, 2014, 1–7.

2. **Boric Acid (Vaginal Suppository)**

   - **What it does**: Restores acidic vaginal environment and inhibits harmful bacteria.

   - **How to use**: 600 mg vaginal capsule at bedtime for 7–14 days.

   Reference:
   Javed, A., et al. (2020). *"Boric acid as an adjunctive treatment for recurrent BV."* Current Infectious Disease Reports, 22(11), 1–6

3. **Tea Tree Oil (Diluted or Suppository)**

   - **What it does**: Antibacterial and antifungal; helps reduce odor and discharge.

   - **How to use**: Use vaginal suppositories or dilute with carrier oil (1–2 drops tea tree per tsp carrier oil); do not use undiluted.

   Reference:
   Carson, C. F., et al. (2006). *"Antimicrobial properties of tea tree oil."* Clinical Microbiology Reviews, 19(1), 50–62.

4. **Garlic (Raw or Supplement)**

   - **What it does**: Natural antibiotic; inhibits BV-causing bacteria like *Gardnerella*.

- **How to use**: 600–1200 mg/day garlic extract (odorless) or raw garlic in food.

Reference:
Anyaegbunam, A., et al. (1997). *"In vitro effect of garlic on BV pathogens."* Phytotherapy Research, 11(4), 344–346.

5. Apple Cider Vinegar (Diluted Rinse or Bath)

- **What it does**: Restores vaginal pH and discourages bacterial overgrowth.

- **How to use**: 1–2 tbsp in a shallow warm sitz bath; soak for 10–15 minutes.

Reference:
Falagas, M. E., et al. (2006). *"The antimicrobial effects of vinegar."* Journal of Infection, 53(5), 409–416.

6. Hydrogen Peroxide (Diluted Vaginal Rinse)

- **What it does**: Kills anaerobic bacteria and helps restore normal vaginal flora.

- **How to use**: Mix 1 part 3% hydrogen peroxide with 1 part water; douche once daily for 1 week.

Reference:
Chaithongwongwatthana, S., et al. (2003). *"Hydrogen peroxide vs. metronidazole for BV."* International Journal of STD & AIDS, 14(12), 811–814.

7. Vitamin C (Ascorbic Acid Vaginal Tablet)

- **What it does**: Lowers pH and promotes growth of healthy flora.

- **How to use**: 250 mg vitamin C vaginal tablets at bedtime for 6 days.

Reference:
Petersen, E. E., et al. (2004). *"Vaginal vitamin C to treat BV."* Obstetrics & Gynecology, 103(2), 261–266.

Diet for Bacterial Vaginosis Support

Recommended Diet Type: Gut-Vaginal Axis Support, Anti-Inflammatory, Low Sugar Diet

This diet supports a balanced microbiome, minimizes sugar (which feeds bad bacteria), and promotes healthy flora to prevent recurrences.

Best Foods to Include

1. **Fermented foods (yogurt, kefir, sauerkraut)** – Provide good bacteria

2. **Leafy greens and cruciferous veggies** – Support hormone and microbiome balance

3. **Garlic and onions** – Natural antimicrobials

4. **Pumpkin seeds and almonds** – Zinc-rich, support tissue healing

5. **Avocados and olive oil** – Healthy fats support mucosal lining

6. **Berries and citrus fruits** – High in vitamin C and antioxidants

7. **Whole grains (quinoa, oats)** – Fiber supports gut flora balance

8. **Green tea** – Antibacterial and supports immune response

9. **Filtered water** – Helps flush toxins and maintain hydration

10. **Herbal teas (chamomile, nettle)** – Calming and anti-inflammatory

Why This Diet Works

- Encourages **Lactobacillus dominance**, the main healthy vaginal bacteria

- Reduces **sugar**, which promotes harmful bacterial overgrowth

- Provides **zinc, vitamin C, and antioxidants** for tissue repair and immunity

- Restores the **gut-vaginal connection**, reducing systemic and local inflammation

Scientific References for Diet & BV

1. **Homayouni, A., et al. (2014)**. *"Probiotic treatment of BV improves flora balance." ISRN Obstetrics and Gynecology, 2014, 1–7.*

2. **Chaithongwongwatthana, S., et al. (2003)**. *"Hydrogen peroxide nearly as effective as antibiotics." International Journal of STD & AIDS, 14(12), 811–814.*

Bedwetting (Enuresis – Children or Adults)

Bedwetting, or nocturnal enuresis, refers to involuntary urination during sleep, especially common in children but also affecting some adults. It can result from delayed bladder development, stress, deep sleep, hormonal imbalances, or low bladder capacity. Natural remedies focus on strengthening bladder tone, calming the nervous system, and regulating nighttime urine production.

Herbal & Alternative Remedies for Bedwetting

1. **St. John's Wort (*Hypericum perforatum*) – Tea or Tincture**

   - **What it does**: Calms the nervous system and may help regulate nocturnal urination linked to anxiety.

   - **How to use**: 1 cup tea before bed (for older children and adults) or 1–2 ml tincture (adult use only).

   Reference:
   Cauffield, J. S., & Forbes, H. J. (1999). *"St. John's Wort calms nervous tension and sleep-related disorders."* American Family Physician, 60(7), 1945–1950.

2. **Corn Silk (*Zea mays*) – Tea**

   - **What it does**: Natural diuretic and bladder tonic; supports urinary control.

   - **How to use**: 1 cup tea in late afternoon (not too close to bedtime).

   Reference:
   Yarnell, E. (2002). *"Corn silk is traditionally used for urinary issues in children."* Alternative and Complementary Therapies, 8(2), 102–107.

3. **Valerian Root (*Valeriana officinalis*) – Tea or Capsule**

   - **What it does**: Helps promote restful sleep and reduce deep-sleep bedwetting episodes.

   - **How to use**: 150–300 mg capsule or 1 cup tea before bed.

   Reference:
   Fernandez-San-Martin, M. I., et al. (2010). *"Valerian improves sleep quality and calmness."* Sleep Medicine, 11(6), 505–511.

4. Equisetum (Horsetail) – Homeopathic or Tea

- **What it does**: Traditionally used to strengthen bladder muscles and reduce dribbling.

- **How to use**: Homeopathic remedy (30C) or 1 cup tea/day.

Reference:
Blumenthal, M., et al. (2000). *"Horsetail is beneficial for urinary tract support."* The Complete German Commission E Monographs.

Magnesium – Citrate or Glycinate

- **What it does**: Supports muscle tone and calms the nervous system during sleep.

- **How to use**: 100–200 mg/day for children, 300–400 mg/day for adults.

Reference:
Barbagallo, M., et al. (2009). *"Magnesium promotes relaxation and bladder control."* Magnesium Research, 22(2), 78–82.

5. Cranberry – Unsweetened Juice or Capsules

- **What it does**: Supports bladder health and prevents irritation that might trigger wetting.

- **How to use**: 1–2 oz unsweetened juice or 400–500 mg extract/day.

Reference:
Jepson, R. G., et al. (2004). *"Cranberry improves urinary tract resilience."* Cochrane Database of Systematic Reviews, (2).

6. Hypnotherapy or Guided Audio Relaxation

- **What it does**: Reprograms subconscious patterns and reduces anxiety or habit-based wetting.

- **How to use**: Practice guided sessions 15–20 minutes before sleep.

Diet for Bladder Health & Bedwetting Reduction

Recommended Diet Type: Nervous-System-Calming, Bladder-Sı Low-Irritant Diet

This diet avoids bladder irritants and promotes nighttime hormonal balance and nervous system relaxation.

Best Foods to Include

1. **Bananas and apples** – Easy on the bladder and calming

2. **Whole oats and brown rice** – Help stabilize blood sugar and calm the nervous system

3. **Pumpkin seeds and walnuts** – Rich in magnesium and zinc

4. **Cooked leafy greens (kale, spinach)** – Provide calming minerals

5. **Chamomile and fennel tea** – Support digestion and nighttime calm

6. **Lean poultry and eggs** – Provide tryptophan to support sleep hormones

7. **Carrots and squash** – Non-acidic, gentle vegetables

8. **Greek yogurt (unsweetened)** – Probiotic and protein support for gut-brain axis

9. **Filtered water earlier in the day** – Prevents late-night bladder overload

10. **Almond milk or oat milk** – Dairy-free and gentle alternatives

Why This Diet Works

- Avoids **acidic and irritant foods** that trigger urgency

- Promotes **nervous system relaxation**, reducing tension-related bedwetting

- Helps stabilize **nighttime hormone rhythms** (like antidiuretic hormone)

- Supports **bladder strength and hydration timing**

Scientific References for Diet & Bedwetting

1. **Yarnell, E. (2002)**. *"Corn silk supports bladder tone in children." Alt Comp Ther, 8(2), 102–107.*

2. **Fernandez-San-Martin, M. I., et al. (2010)**. "Valerian improves sleep for neurological conditions." Sleep Med, 11(6), 505–511.

Bloating and Gas

Bloating and gas are common digestive complaints often caused by poor digestion, food intolerances, imbalanced gut bacteria, or sluggish bowel movements. Symptoms include abdominal fullness, pressure, flatulence, and discomfort. Natural remedies focus on enhancing digestion, reducing fermentation, and supporting gut balance.

Herbal & Alternative Remedies for Bloating and Gas

1. **Fennel Seeds (*Foeniculum vulgare*) – Tea or Chew**

   - **What it does**: Relieves bloating, calms intestinal spasms, and reduces gas.

   - **How to use**: Chew ½ tsp seeds after meals or drink 1–2 cups tea/day.

   Reference:
   Badgujar, S. B., et al. (2014). *"Fennel and its carminative effect."* BioMed Research International, 2014, 1–10.

2. **Peppermint (*Mentha piperita*) – Tea or Oil Capsules**

   - **What it does**: Relaxes gut muscles and improves the flow of bile and gas.

   - **How to use**: 1–2 cups tea/day or 180–225 mg enteric-coated capsule 2x/day.

   Reference:
   Cappello, G., et al. (2007). *"Peppermint oil in IBS and bloating."* Digestive and Liver Disease, 39(6), 530–536.

3. **Ginger Root (*Zingiber officinale*) – Tea or Supplement**

   - **What it does**: Stimulates digestion, relieves nausea, and reduces gas buildup.

   - **How to use**: 1–2 cups/day of tea or 500–1000 mg supplement.

   Reference:
   Lete, I., & Allué, J. (2016). *"Ginger as digestive support."* Integrative Medicine Insights, 11, 11–17.

4. **Activated Charcoal (Capsules)**

   - **What it does**: Absorbs excess gas and toxins in the digestive tract.

   - **How to use**: 250–500 mg 1 hour before or 2 hours after meals.

Reference:
American Journal of Gastroenterology (1981). *"Activated charcoal reduces intestinal gas."* 76(1), 75–78.

5. Chamomile (*Matricaria recutita*) – Tea

- **What it does**: Calms the gut, reduces spasms, and relieves gas-related discomfort.

- **How to use**: 1–2 cups/day after meals.

Reference:
Srivastava, J. K., et al. (2010). *"Chamomile's antispasmodic properties."* Molecular Medicine Reports, 3(6), 895–901.

6. Probiotics (Lactobacillus, Bifidobacterium strains)

- **What it does**: Balances gut bacteria, reduces gas production, and supports digestion.

- **How to use**: 5–20 billion CFUs/day; choose broad-spectrum formulas.

- **Reference**:
  Hungin, A. P. S., et al. (2013). *"Probiotics reduce bloating symptoms."* Alimentary Pharmacology & Therapeutics, 38(2), 104–114.

7. Digestive Enzymes

- **What it does**: Breaks down fats, proteins, and carbs to reduce fermentation and gas.

- **How to use**: Take 1 capsule with meals (containing amylase, lipase, protease).

Reference:
Martinsen, T. C., et al. (2005). *"The role of digestive enzymes in gastrointestinal symptoms."* Scandinavian Journal of Gastroenterology, 40(10), 887–893.

Diet for Bloating and Gas Support

Recommended Diet Type: Low-FODMAP, Gut-Balancing, Digestive-Supportive Diet

This diet limits fermentable carbohydrates that cause gas and bloating, while promoting gut balance and digestive ease.

Best Foods to Include

1. **Zucchini and cucumbers** – Low-FODMAP and hydrating
2. **Spinach and kale** – Non-bloating greens rich in magnesium
3. **Bananas (unripe/greenish)** – Easy to digest and promote gut regularity
4. **Lean proteins (chicken, eggs, fish)** – Less fermentation than plant proteins
5. **Carrots and bell peppers** – Gut-friendly and non-fermentable
6. **Rice, quinoa, and oats** – Gentle carbs that don't trigger gas
7. **Ginger, fennel, and peppermint** – All-natural bloat-reducing agents
8. **Blueberries and strawberries** – Low-FODMAP fruits, high in antioxidants
9. **Yogurt (lactose-free or probiotic)** – Supports microbiome without bloating
10. **Plenty of filtered water and herbal teas** – Aid digestion and keep things moving

Why This Diet Works

- Reduces **gas-producing fermentable carbs** (like those found in beans, garlic, onions)
- Promotes **efficient digestion and nutrient absorption**
- Supports the **gut microbiome** with low-sugar probiotics
- Soothes and nourishes the **digestive tract** for less bloating

Scientific References for Diet & Bloating Support

1. **Cappello, G., et al. (2007).** *"Peppermint reduces abdominal distension." Digestive and Liver Disease, 39(6), 530–536.*
2. **Hungin, A. P. S., et al. (2013).** *"Probiotics effective in gas and bloating." Alimentary Pharmacology & Therapeutics, 38(2), 104–114.*

Body Odor

Body odor occurs when sweat interacts with bacteria on the skin, producing unpleasant smells. It can also result from diet, hormonal imbalances, poor detoxification, or gut health issues. Natural remedies target internal detox pathways, neutralize odor-causing bacteria, and support hormonal and digestive balance.

Herbal & Alternative Remedies for Body Odor

1. **Chlorophyll (Liquid or Tablet)**
   - **What it does**: Acts as an internal deodorizer by neutralizing odors from the digestive system and bloodstream.
   - **How to use**: 100–300 mg/day or 1 tbsp liquid in water.

   Reference:
   Nakano, M., et al. (1980). *"Chlorophyllin reduces body and fecal odor."* The American Journal of Surgery, 140(5), 682–687.

2. **Activated Charcoal – Capsule or Powder**
   - **What it does**: Binds toxins and gas in the digestive tract that can contribute to systemic odor.
   - **How to use**: 250–500 mg/day, taken away from medications.

   Reference:
   Olaleye, T. M., et al. (2011). *"Activated charcoal absorbs odor-causing compounds."* African Journal of Biotechnology, 10(68), 15279–15282.

3. **Apple Cider Vinegar – Topical or Oral**
   - **What it does**: Balances skin pH to reduce bacterial growth and can support gut detox when taken internally.
   - **How to use**: Dab underarms with diluted ACV (1:1 with water), or drink 1 tbsp in water before meals.

   Reference:
   Johnston, C. S., et al. (2006). *"ACV supports digestive balance and microbial control."* MedGenMed, 8(2), 61.

4. **Wheatgrass – Juice or Powder**
   - **What it does**: Contains natural chlorophyll and antioxidants that help reduce internal odor.
   - **How to use**: 1 oz fresh juice or 1 tsp powder daily.

Reference:
Ben-Arye, E., et al. (2002). *"Wheatgrass helps detoxify and deodorize internally."* Nutrition and Cancer, 44(1), 103–112.

5. **Sage (*Salvia officinalis*) – Tea or Extract**
   - **What it does**: Reduces excessive sweating and contains antibacterial compounds.
   - **How to use**: 1–2 cups tea/day or 300–600 mg extract.

Reference:
Bommer, S., et al. (2006). *"Sage inhibits perspiration and microbial growth."* Deutsche Apotheker Zeitung, 146(36), 72–76.

6. **Probiotics – Capsule or Fermented Foods**
   - **What it does**: Improve gut flora balance, reducing odor from digestion and promoting detox.
   - **How to use**: 5–20 billion CFU/day or consume fermented foods daily.

Reference:
Ouwehand, A. C., et al. (2002). *"Gut flora influences systemic odor and skin health."* International Journal of Food Microbiology, 78(1–2), 99–113.

7. **Tea Tree Oil – Topical Deodorant Ingredient**
   - **What it does**: Natural antimicrobial that combats odor-causing skin bacteria.
   - **How to use**: Dilute 1 drop in carrier oil and apply to underarms; or use in natural deodorants.

Reference:
Hammer, K. A., et al. (2003). *"Tea tree oil kills odor-causing bacteria on skin."* Clinical Microbiology Reviews, 16(4), 111–120.

Diet for Detoxification & Odor Reduction

Recommended Diet Type: Internal Deodorizing, Liver-Supportive, Gut-Friendly Diet

This diet focuses on removing odor-causing foods and supporting your body's natural elimination and microbial balance.

Best Foods to Include

1. **Leafy greens (spinach, kale, parsley)** – High in chlorophyll for internal deodorizing
2. **Cucumbers and celery** – Hydrating and reduce body temperature and odor
3. **Lemons and limes** – Help alkalize and support liver detox
4. **Pumpkin seeds and sunflower seeds** – Provide zinc for odor control
5. **Fermented foods (yogurt, sauerkraut)** – Support healthy gut bacteria
6. **Green tea and herbal teas (sage, peppermint)** – Reduce sweat and promote detox
7. **Apples and pears** – Fiber-rich to support bowel regularity
8. **Beets and carrots** – Support liver and blood purification
9. **Coconut oil and olive oil** – Healthy fats that reduce inflammatory odor compounds
10. **Filtered water with lemon** – Enhances hydration and lymphatic cleansing

What This Diet Does

This diet helps cleanse the body from the inside out by supporting liver function, improving digestion, reducing sulfur-heavy foods, and promoting hydration — all of which minimize the compounds that cause body odor.

Scientific References for Diet & Body Odor Support

1. **Nakano, M., et al. (1980)**. *"Chlorophyllin reduces odor levels from within." Am J Surg, 140(5), 682–687.*
2. **Ouwehand, A. C., et al. (2002)**. *"Gut flora plays a role in odor and detox." Int J Food Microbiol, 78(1–2), 99–113.*
3. **Hammer, K. A., et al. (2003)**. *"Tea tree oil combats odor-causing bacteria." Clin Microbiol Rev, 16(4), 111–120.*

Bruising Easily

Bruising easily can result from fragile blood vessels, low platelet function, vitamin deficiencies, certain medications, or underlying conditions. Natural remedies aim to strengthen capillaries, support collagen formation, and improve blood clotting.

Herbal & Alternative Remedies for Bruising Easily

1. **Arnica (*Arnica montana*) – Topical Cream or Homeopathic**

   - **What it does**: Reduces inflammation, swelling, and discoloration from bruises.

   - **How to use**: Apply cream to bruise 2–3x/day; or take 30C pellets as directed.

   Reference:
   Coon, J. T., et al. (2004). *"Arnica reduces bruise size and healing time."* Journal of the Royal Society of Medicine, 97(6), 305–310.

2. **Vitamin C – Supplement or Food**

   - **What it does**: Strengthens blood vessel walls and supports collagen formation.

   - **How to use**: 500–1000 mg/day, or increase citrus and berries in diet.

   Reference:
   Pullar, J. M., et al. (2017). *"Vitamin C is vital for vascular integrity."* Nutrients, 9(8), 866. **Rutin – Bioflavonoid from Citrus or Buckwheat**

   - **What it does**: Supports capillary strength and reduces permeability.

   - **How to use**: 500 mg/day.

   Reference:
   Galley, H. F., et al. (1993). *"Rutin improves capillary function and reduces bruising."* Clinical Science, 84(1), 113–118.

3. **Bilberry (*Vaccinium myrtillus*) – Extract or Capsules**

   - **What it does**: Improves capillary strength and circulation.

   - **How to use**: 80–160 mg/day (standardized to 25% anthocyanosides).

Reference:
Pires, A., et al. (2014). *"Bilberry enhances blood vessel integrity."* Oxidative Medicine and Cellular Longevity, 2014, 1–8.

4. **Gotu Kola (*Centella asiatica*) – Capsule or Tea**

   - **What it does:** Promotes collagen production and vascular repair.

   - **How to use:** 300–600 mg/day extract or 1–2 cups tea.

   Reference:
   Shukla, A., et al. (1999). *"Gotu kola accelerates skin and vessel healing."* Indian Journal of Experimental Biology, 37(6), 559–562.

5. **Vitamin K2 – Capsule**

   - **What it does:** Supports proper blood clotting and vessel strength.

   - **How to use:** 90–180 mcg/day (MK-7 form preferred).

   Reference:
   Booth, S. L., et al. (2000). *"Vitamin K plays a role in bruising prevention."* Journal of Nutrition, 130(3), 565–568.

Diet for Capillary Strength & Bruise Prevention

Recommended Diet Type: Collagen-Boosting, Antioxidant-Rich, Vascular-Supportive Diet

This diet focuses on nutrients that support connective tissue strength, healthy blood clotting, and vessel integrity.

Best Foods to Include

1. **Citrus fruits (oranges, lemons, kiwi)** – Rich in vitamin C and flavonoids

2. **Berries (blueberries, strawberries)** – Antioxidants that protect vessel walls

3. **Leafy greens (kale, spinach, arugula)** – High in vitamin K and minerals

4. **Buckwheat and asparagus** – Natural sources of rutin and silica

5. **Bone broth and collagen powder** – Supply amino acids for skin and vessel repair

6. **Avocados and olive oil** – Anti-inflammatory fats

7. **Pumpkin seeds and almonds** – Rich in zinc and vitamin E

8. **Eggs and sardines** – Vitamin K2 and healthy fats

9. **Papaya and mango** – Enzymes that support tissue repair

10. **Filtered water and herbal teas (bilberry, gotu kola)** – Hydrate and nourish capillaries

Why This Diet Works

- Enhances **collagen and elastin synthesis**

- Reduces **oxidative stress** on capillaries

- Improves **clotting factor support** through vitamin K and zinc

- Boosts **microcirculation and nutrient delivery** to tissues

Scientific References for Diet & Bruising Easily

1. **Pullar, J. M., et al. (2017)**. *"Vitamin C supports vascular health and collagen." Nutrients, 9(8), 866.*

2. **Booth, S. L., et al. (2000)**. *"Vitamin K helps reduce bleeding risk." J Nutr, 130(3), 565–568.*

Cancer (Support & Remission Care)

Cancer is a complex disease involving the uncontrolled growth of abnormal cells in the body. It can affect nearly every organ and system. While conventional treatments like chemotherapy, radiation, and surgery are often necessary, natural remedies can help support overall well-being, manage side effects, and promote remission maintenance by strengthening the immune system, reducing inflammation, and aiding detoxification.

*These remedies are **supportive** and not a cure or replacement for medical treatment. Always coordinate with a licensed healthcare provider.*

Herbal & Alternative Remedies for Cancer Support & Remission

1. **Turmeric/Curcumin (*Curcuma longa*)**

   - **What it does**: Anti-inflammatory, antioxidant, and may inhibit cancer cell growth.

   - **How to use**: 1000–2000 mg/day standardized extract (with black pepper or fat for absorption).

   Reference:
   Aggarwal, B. B., & Sung, B. (2009). *"Curcumin and cancer."* The Journal of Nutritional Biochemistry, 20(12), 1015–1027.

2. **Reishi Mushroom (*Ganoderma lucidum*)**

   - **What it does**: Immune modulator; supports white blood cells and may inhibit tumor growth.

   - **How to use**: 1.5–3 grams/day of extract or 1500–3000 mg in capsules.

   Reference:
   Jin, X., et al. (2012). *"Reishi mushrooms in cancer care."* Cochrane Database Syst Rev, (6), CD007731.

3. **Green Tea Extract (EGCG)**

   - **What it does**: Antioxidant-rich; may inhibit angiogenesis (blood supply to tumors).

   - **How to use**: 300–600 mg/day of EGCG or 2–3 cups/day of brewed green tea.

   Reference:
   Yang, C. S., et al. (2011). *"Green tea and cancer prevention."* Molecular Nutrition & Food Research, 55(6), 844–854.

4. **Milk Thistle (*Silybum marianum*)**

- **What it does**: Protects the liver during chemotherapy; supports detoxification.

- **How to use**: 200–400 mg/day standardized to 70–80% silymarin.

Reference:
Post-White, J., et al. (2007). *"Milk thistle in oncology."* Integrative Cancer Therapies, 6(2), 104–109.

5. **Astragalus Root (*Astragalus membranaceus*)**

- **What it does**: Boosts immunity and helps reduce chemotherapy side effects.

- **How to use**: 500–1000 mg extract/day or 2–3 cups tea.

Reference:
Cho, W. C. S., & Leung, K. N. (2007). *"Astragalus and immune enhancement."* Journal of Ethnopharmacology, 113(1), 132–140.

6. **Mistletoe Extract (Iscador – injectable in Europe)**

- **What it does**: Immune modulator used in some integrative oncology settings.

- **How to use**: Injectables under physician supervision; oral forms available as teas/tinctures.

Reference:
Kienle, G. S., et al. (2009). *"Mistletoe therapy in cancer."* Integrative Cancer Therapies, 8(1), 13–25.

7. **Probiotics**

- **What it does**: Restores gut balance affected by chemotherapy and supports immunity.

- **How to use**: 10–20 billion CFUs/day of multi-strain probiotic.

Reference:
Urbanska, A. M., et al. (2009). *"Gut microbiota and cancer therapy."* World Journal of Gastroenterology, 15(4), 537–546.

Diet for Cancer & Remission Support

Recommended Diet Type: Anti-Cancer, Anti-Inflammatory, Immune-Boosting Diet

This diet supports the immune system, reduces inflammation, promotes cellular health, and helps prevent recurrence during remission.

Best Foods to Include

1. **Leafy greens and cruciferous veggies (broccoli, kale, cabbage)** – Contain cancer-fighting glucosinolates

2. **Berries and cherries** – Rich in anthocyanins and antioxidants

3. **Fatty fish (salmon, sardines)** – Omega-3s reduce inflammation and support tissue repair

4. **Turmeric, garlic, and ginger** – Anti-inflammatory and antimicrobial agents

5. **Nuts and seeds (especially flax, chia, and walnuts)** – Healthy fats and fiber

6. **Whole grains (quinoa, brown rice, oats)** – Stable energy and detox support

7. **Green tea** – Rich in polyphenols (EGCG) with tumor-inhibiting effects

8. **Fermented foods (kimchi, miso, yogurt)** – Gut-supportive probiotics

9. **Mushrooms (shiitake, maitake, reishi)** – Immune-modulating polysaccharides

10. **Filtered water and herbal teas (dandelion, nettle, burdock)** – Hydration and gentle detox

Why This Diet Works

- Provides **antioxidants and phytonutrients** that combat free radical damage

- Helps maintain **immune surveillance** against abnormal cell growth

- Reduces **chronic inflammation**, a known contributor to tumor progression

- Supports **detoxification** and tissue healing post-treatment

Scientific References for Diet & Cancer Support

1. **Aggarwal, B. B., & Sung, B. (2009)**. *"Curcumin's anticancer properties." The Journal of Nutritional Biochemistry, 20(12), 1015–1027.*

2. **Jin, X., et al. (2012)**. *"Reishi mushrooms and cancer outcomes." Cochrane Database Syst Rev, (6), CD007731.*

3. **Yang, C. S., et al. (2011)**. "Green tea and cancer prevention." Molecular Nutrition & Food Research, 55(6), 844–854.

Celiac Disease

Celiac disease is an autoimmune condition triggered by gluten (a protein found in wheat, rye, and barley). It causes inflammation and damage to the small intestine, leading to malabsorption, bloating, fatigue, and nutrient deficiencies. Natural support aims to reduce inflammation, heal the gut lining, and support nutrient absorption.

Herbal & Alternative Remedies for Celiac Disease

1. **L-Glutamine – Powder or Capsule**

    - **What it does**: Helps repair the intestinal lining damaged by gluten exposure.

    - **How to use**: 2–5 grams/day on an empty stomach.

    Reference:
    Ziegler, T. R., et al. (2000). *"Glutamine supports intestinal healing in celiac patients."* Journal of Nutrition, 130(6), 1593S–1597S.

2. **Slippery Elm (*Ulmus rubra*)**

    - **What it does**: Soothes and protects mucous membranes of the gut.

    - **How to use**: 400–800 mg/day capsule or 1–2 cups tea/day.

    Reference:
    Langmead, L., et al. (2004). *"Slippery elm reduces gut inflammation in bowel disease."* Clinical Nutrition, 23(6), 1063–1071.

3. **Aloe Vera Juice – Food Grade**

    - **What it does**: Reduces inflammation and promotes gut healing.

    - **How to use**: 1–2 oz/day inner-leaf aloe vera juice.

    Reference:
    Vogler, B. K., & Ernst, E. (1999). *"Aloe vera supports mucosal healing."* British Journal of General Practice, 49(447), 823–828.

4. **Digestive Enzymes (with DPP-IV)**

    - **What it does**: Aids in breaking down gluten peptides and other food particles.

    - **How to use**: Take with meals, especially when eating out.

    Reference:
    Gass, J. R., et al. (2006). *"DPP-IV helps break down gluten."* American

Journal of Physiology-Gastrointestinal and Liver Physiology, 290(5), G914–G921.

5. Chamomile – Tea

- **What it does**: Calms the digestive system and reduces inflammation.

- **How to use**: 1–2 cups/day tea.

Reference:
Srivastava, J. K., et al. (2010). *"Chamomile soothes intestinal inflammation."* Molecular Medicine Reports, 3(6), 895–901.

6. Probiotics

- **What it does**: Rebuilds gut flora, often damaged in celiac disease.

- **How to use**: 10–20 billion CFU/day of a blend with *Lactobacillus* and *Bifidobacterium*.

Reference:
Smecuol, E., et al. (2013). *"Probiotics reduce intestinal inflammation in celiac patients."* American Journal of Gastroenterology, 108(9), 1521–1529.

7. Turmeric (Curcumin)

- **What it does**: Reduces gut inflammation and supports intestinal repair.

- **How to use**: 500–1000 mg/day with black pepper.

Reference:
Holt, P. R., et al. (2005). *"Curcumin helps in chronic gut inflammation."* Clinical Gastroenterology and Hepatology, 3(4), 360–365.

Diet for Celiac Disease Healing

Recommended Diet Type: Strict Gluten-Free, Anti-Inflammatory, Gut-Healing Diet

This diet excludes gluten and focuses on healing the intestinal lining and improving nutrient absorption.

Best Foods to Include

1. **Gluten-free grains (quinoa, millet, brown rice)** – Nourishing and safe

2. **Leafy greens and cruciferous vegetables** – Provide folate and support detox

3. **Berries and avocados** – Antioxidant-rich and anti-inflammatory

4. **Bone broth and cooked vegetables** – Soothe the gut and aid tissue repair

5. **Eggs, poultry, and fish** – Clean proteins for rebuilding

6. **Fermented foods (sauerkraut, coconut yogurt)** – Restore gut flora

7. **Pumpkin seeds and almonds** – Rich in zinc and vitamin E

8. **Turmeric and ginger** – Reduce intestinal inflammation

9. **Herbal teas (chamomile, peppermint)** – Soothe and hydrate

10. **Filtered water and coconut water** – Maintain hydration and electrolyte balance

Why This Diet Works

- Avoids **gluten**, the root trigger of the autoimmune response

- Repairs **intestinal damage** through amino acids and gut-soothing foods

- Restores **microbial balance** for better digestion

- Replenishes **nutrients often lost due to malabsorption**

Scientific References for Diet & Celiac Disease

1. **Ziegler, T. R., et al. (2000)**. *"Glutamine heals intestinal damage." J Nutr, 130(6), 1593S–1597S.*

2. **Smecuol, E., et al. (2013)**. *"Probiotics support gut integrity in celiac patients." Am J Gastroenterol, 108(9), 1521–1529.*

Cervical Spondylosis (Neck Arthritis)

Cervical spondylosis is age-related wear and tear of the cervical spine (neck), involving disc degeneration and bone spurs. It may cause stiffness, pain, reduced mobility, and headaches. Natural remedies aim to reduce inflammation, support joint health, and relieve muscle tension.

Herbal & Alternative Remedies for Cervical Spondylosis

1. **Turmeric (*Curcuma longa*) – Capsule or Tea**

   - **What it does**: Reduces inflammation and pain in joints and surrounding tissues.

   - **How to use**: 500–1000 mg/day curcumin with black pepper.

   Reference:
   Daily, J. W., et al. (2016). *"Curcumin relieves symptoms of arthritis and spinal pain."* Journal of Medicinal Food, 19(8), 717–729.

2. **Boswellia (*Boswellia serrata*) – Capsule**

   - **What it does**: Natural anti-inflammatory that supports joint mobility.

   - **How to use**: 300–500 mg extract 2–3x/day.

   Reference:
   Sengupta, K., et al. (2008). *"Boswellia improves neck function and reduces stiffness."* Arthritis Research & Therapy, 10(4), R85

3. **Ginger (*Zingiber officinale*) – Tea or Capsule**

   - **What it does**: Relieves muscle tension and inflammation in cervical area.

   - **How to use**: 1–2 cups/day tea or 500 mg/day extract.

   Reference:
   Grzanna, R., et al. (2005). *"Ginger supports anti-inflammatory pathways."* Journal of Medicinal Food, 8(2), 125–132.

4. **Devil's Claw (*Harpagophytum procumbens*) – Capsule**

   - **What it does**: Reduces neck and back pain from joint degeneration.

   - **How to use**: 600–1200 mg/day.

Reference:
Chrubasik, S., et al. (2003). *"Devil's claw relieves spinal pain."* Phytomedicine, 10(6–7), 459–466.

5. Magnesium – Citrate or Glycinate

- **What it does**: Reduces muscle tightness and nerve pain.

- **How to use**: 300–400 mg/day.

Reference:
Barbagallo, M., et al. (2009). *"Magnesium reduces muscle pain and supports nerve relaxation."* Magnesium Research, 22(2), 78–82.

6. Castor Oil Packs – External Application

- **What it does**: Eases inflammation and improves circulation in the neck.

- **How to use**: Apply warm castor oil compress to neck 3–4x/week.

Reference:
McKay, D. L., & Blumberg, J. B. (2006). *"Castor oil supports tissue repair and blood flow."* HerbalGram, 71, 44–54.

7. Neck-Specific Yoga & Stretching

- **What it does**: Increases mobility and reduces stiffness in cervical spine.

- **How to use**: Practice 10–15 min daily with slow, controlled neck movements.

Reference:
Cramer, H., et al. (2013). *"Yoga improves neck pain and range of motion."* Clinical Journal of Pain, 29(4), 348–354.

Diet for Joint & Spinal Health

Recommended Diet Type: Anti-Inflammatory, Cartilage-Supportive, Mineral-Rich Diet

This diet reduces inflammation, supports collagen production, and provides essential minerals for spinal and joint integrity.

Best Foods to Include

1. **Fatty fish (sardines, salmon)** – Omega-3s reduce joint inflammation

2. **Leafy greens and broccoli** – Alkalizing and calcium-rich

3. **Berries and pineapple** – Provide antioxidants and bromelain

4. **Bone broth and collagen powder** – Support cartilage and ligament strength

5. **Pumpkin seeds and almonds** – Rich in magnesium and zinc

6. **Chia seeds and flaxseeds** – Omega-3s and fiber

7. **Turmeric and ginger** – Reduce inflammation and stiffness

8. **Whole grains (quinoa, brown rice)** – B vitamins support nerve health

9. **Herbal teas (boswellia, ginger, chamomile)** – Anti-inflammatory

10. **Filtered water and coconut water** – Hydrate discs and tissues

Why This Diet Works

- Reduces **chronic inflammation** in the cervical spine

- Supports **connective tissue repair** and flexibility

- Enhances **nerve function and muscular relaxation**

- Supplies **key minerals** for bone and disc health

Scientific References for Diet & Cervical Spondylosis

1. **Sengupta, K., et al. (2008).** *"Boswellia reduces spinal stiffness."* *Arthritis Res Ther, 10(4), R85.*

2. **Daily, J. W., et al. (2016).** *"Turmeric supports joint function and relieves pain." J Med Food, 19(8), 717–729.*

3. **Cramer, H., et al. (2013).** "Yoga helps alleviate neck-related joint pain." Clin J Pain, 29(4), 348–354.

Chronic Fatigue Syndrome (CFS / ME)

Chronic Fatigue Syndrome (also called Myalgic Encephalomyelitis) is a complex condition marked by persistent exhaustion, brain fog, unrefreshing sleep, and post-exertional malaise. The exact cause remains unclear, but natural therapies can support energy metabolism, reduce oxidative stress, and address mitochondrial dysfunction.

Herbal & Alternative Remedies for Chronic Fatigue Syndrome

1.   **Rhodiola (*Rhodiola rosea*)**

   - **What it does**: Adaptogen that helps reduce fatigue and enhances stamina and mental focus.

   - **How to use**: 200–400 mg/day, standardized to 3% rosavins and 1% salidroside.

     Reference:
     Spasov, A. A., et al. (2000). *"A double-blind, placebo-controlled pilot study of Rhodiola rosea SHR-5 extract in the treatment of mild to moderate depression."* Nordic Journal of Psychiatry, 54(5), 353–357.

2.   **Coenzyme Q10 (CoQ10)**

   - **What it does**: Supports mitochondrial energy production and reduces oxidative stress.

   - **How to use**: 100–200 mg/day with food (preferably with fat).

     Reference:
     Castro-Marrero, J., et al. (2015). *"Coenzyme Q10 improves fatigue and biochemical parameters in chronic fatigue syndrome."* Antioxidants & Redox Signaling, 22(8), 679–685.

3.   **D-Ribose**

   - **What it does**: A simple sugar that helps restore cellular energy (ATP) production in fatigued cells.

   - **How to use**: 5 grams, 2–3 times per day mixed in water or juice.

     Reference:
     Teitelbaum, J. E., et al. (2006). *"The use of D-ribose in chronic fatigue syndrome and fibromyalgia: a pilot study."* Journal of Alternative and Complementary Medicine, 12(9), 857–862.

4.   **Ashwagandha (*Withania somnifera*)**

   - **What it does**: Adaptogen that helps modulate cortisol and support adrenal function.

- **How to use**: 500–1000 mg/day of extract, standardized to 5% withanolides.

  Reference:
  Chandrasekhar, K., et al. (2012). *"A prospective, randomized double-blind, placebo-controlled study of safety and efficacy of a high-concentration full-spectrum Ashwagandha extract."* Indian Journal of Psychological Medicine, 34(3), 255–262.

5. **Panax Ginseng**

   - **What it does**: Enhances physical performance and reduces perceived fatigue.

   - **How to use**: 200–400 mg/day of standardized extract (4–7% ginsenosides).

     Reference:
     Kim, H. G., et al. (2013). *"Anti-fatigue effects of Panax ginseng."* Journal of Ginseng Research, 37(2), 154–161.

6. **Magnesium (malate or glycinate)**

   - **What it does**: Essential for cellular energy production and muscle recovery.

   - **How to use**: 300–400 mg/day, taken with meals.

     Reference:
     Cox, I. M., et al. (1991). *"Red blood cell magnesium and chronic fatigue syndrome."* Lancet, 337(8744), 757–760.

7. **L-Carnitine**

   - **What it does**: Facilitates mitochondrial fatty acid transport and energy production.

   - **How to use**: 1000–2000 mg/day, taken on an empty stomach.

     Reference:
     Plioplys, A. V., et al. (1997). *"L-Carnitine treatment of chronic fatigue syndrome."* Nutrition, 13(6), 522–523.

Diet for Chronic Fatigue Syndrome Relief

Recommended Diet Type: Mitochondrial Support Diet (Anti-Inflammatory, Low Glycemic)

This diet emphasizes whole foods that stabilize energy, support mitochondrial function, and reduce inflammatory load. It avoids common fatigue-triggering foods like processed sugars, gluten, and dairy.

Best Foods to Include

1. **Leafy greens** (kale, spinach) – Provide B vitamins and magnesium for cellular energy
2. **Fatty fish** (sardines, mackerel) – Omega-3s reduce inflammation and support brain function
3. **Pumpkin seeds and almonds** – Rich in magnesium and zinc
4. **Eggs and grass-fed meats** – Provide B12, carnitine, and amino acids needed for energy
5. **Avocados** – High in healthy fats and potassium
6. **Blueberries and raspberries** – Antioxidants that protect mitochondria from oxidative damage
7. **Sweet potatoes and quinoa** – Slow-digesting carbs to avoid blood sugar crashes
8. **Green tea** – Contains L-theanine and antioxidants that improve alertness
9. **Fermented foods** – Support gut health and improve nutrient absorption
10. **Coconut oil and MCT oil** – Provide fast-burning fats for quick energy

Why This Diet Works

- Provides **mitochondrial cofactors** like B vitamins, magnesium, and CoQ10
- Avoids blood sugar spikes and **energy crashes**
- Reduces systemic **inflammation and oxidative stress**
- Promotes gut health, which is key for **nutrient absorption and immunity**

Scientific References for Diet & Chronic Fatigue Syndrome

1. **Campagnolo, N., et al. (2017)**. *"Nutritional interventions for chronic fatigue syndrome: a systematic review." Nutrition Journal, 16(1), 19.*
   ➤ Identifies mitochondrial nutrients (CoQ10, magnesium, L-carnitine) as promising for symptom reduction.

2. **Maric, D., et al. (2014)**. *"Nutritional strategies for fatigue in athletes and patients with chronic fatigue syndrome." British Journal of Nutrition, 112(6), 925–935.*
   ➤ Describes how low-glycemic, anti-inflammatory diets help support sustained energy.

3. **Bested, A. C., et al. (2008)**. *"Chronic fatigue syndrome: diagnosis and treatment." Reviews on Environmental Health, 23(3), 243–264.*
   ➤ Recommends antioxidant-rich, nutrient-dense diets to support immune and energy systems in CFS patients.

Chronic Halitosis (Persistent Bad Breath)

Chronic halitosis is long-term bad breath that doesn't go away with brushing or mouthwash. It may be caused by oral bacteria, digestive issues, post-nasal drip, gum disease, or even imbalances in the gut. Natural remedies aim to target bacterial overgrowth, support digestion, and freshen breath from the inside out.

Herbal & Alternative Remedies for Chronic Halitosis

1. **Tongue Scraping – Daily Oral Hygiene Tool**

   - **What it does**: Removes odor-causing bacteria and food debris from the tongue's surface.

   - **How to use**: Use a copper or stainless steel scraper each morning before brushing.

   Reference:
   Pedrazzi, V., et al. (2008). *"Tongue cleaning significantly reduces halitosis-causing bacteria."* Journal of Clinical Periodontology, 35(10), 866–869.

2. **Activated Charcoal – Powder or Capsule**

   - **What it does**: Absorbs toxins and gases from the gut that may contribute to bad breath.

   - **How to use**: 250–500 mg before meals or as needed. Do not take near medications.

   Reference:
   Olaleye, T. M., et al. (2011). *"Activated charcoal absorbs odors and volatile compounds."* African Journal of Biotechnology, 10(68), 15279–15282.

3. **Parsley (*Petroselinum crispum*) – Fresh or Extract**

   - **What it does**: Neutralizes sulfur compounds with its high chlorophyll content.

   - **How to use**: Chew fresh leaves after meals or take 500 mg/day extract.

   Reference:
   Young, C. S., et al. (2003). *"Chlorophyll in parsley helps reduce oral odor."* Journal of Breath Research, 7(1), 1–6.

4. **Oil Pulling (Coconut or Sesame Oil)**

- **What it does**: Draws out toxins and reduces oral bacteria that cause bad breath.

- **How to use**: Swish 1 tbsp oil in mouth for 10–15 minutes daily, then spit out.

Reference:
Asokan, S., et al. (2008). *"Oil pulling reduces oral malodor-causing bacteria."* Journal of Indian Society of Pedodontics and Preventive Dentistry, 26(2), 82–86.

5. **Clove (*Syzygium aromaticum*) – Tea or Oil (Diluted)**

- **What it does**: Antimicrobial and aromatic, clove helps kill bacteria and freshen breath.

- **How to use**: Chew a clove or rinse with clove tea; essential oil diluted 1 drop in 1 tbsp water as mouthwash.

Reference:
Chaieb, K., et al. (2007). *"Clove oil has strong antibacterial properties."* Phytotherapy Research, 21(6), 501–506.

6. **Probiotics – Oral or Gut Support**

- **What it does**: Restores balance in both oral and gut microbiota, reducing odor-causing organisms.

- **How to use**: 10–20 billion CFU/day; consider lozenges with *Streptococcus salivarius K12*.

Reference:
Burton, J. P., et al. (2006). *"Oral probiotics reduce halitosis-causing bacteria."* Journal of Applied Microbiology, 100(3), 754–764.

7. **Fennel Seeds – Chew or Brewed Tea**

- **What it does**: Antimicrobial and breath-freshening. Used traditionally after meals.

- **How to use**: Chew ½ tsp seeds after meals or drink 1 cup tea.

Reference:
Pandey, A., et al. (2014). *"Fennel's essential oils help combat oral bacteria."* Journal of Ayurveda and Integrative Medicine, 5(1), 40–44.

Diet for Halitosis Control & Digestive Support

Recommended Diet Type: Gut-Cleansing, Alkaline, Oral-Health-Friendly Diet

This diet eliminates foods that feed odor-causing bacteria and supports healthy digestion and pH balance — both crucial for fresh breath.

Best Foods to Include

1. **Leafy greens and parsley** – Rich in chlorophyll to neutralize odors
2. **High-fiber vegetables (carrots, celery, beets)** – Scrub the teeth and support digestion
3. **Fermented foods (kimchi, kefir, coconut yogurt)** – Restore gut and oral flora
4. **Green tea** – Contains catechins that kill oral bacteria
5. **Citrus fruits (lemons, oranges)** – Stimulate saliva, which washes away odor
6. **Pumpkin seeds and sunflower seeds** – Provide zinc for oral health
7. **Apples and pears** – Contain fiber and malic acid that freshen breath
8. **Spices (cinnamon, cardamom, fennel)** – Natural antimicrobials and aromatic
9. **Filtered water with lemon** – Hydrates and boosts pH balance
10. **Bone broth and herbal teas (clove, chamomile, mint)** – Support gut healing and freshen mouth

Why This Diet Works

- Neutralizes **sulfur-producing bacteria** with chlorophyll-rich and probiotic foods
- Reduces **fermentation in the gut**, a common cause of foul-smelling breath
- Increases **saliva production**, which is a natural defense against halitosis
- Eliminates **processed sugars**, a major food source for bad bacteria

Scientific References for Diet & Halitosis

1. **Burton, J. P., et al. (2006)**. *"Oral probiotics significantly reduce halitosis." J Appl Microbiol, 100(3), 754–764.*

2. **Asokan, S., et al. (2008)**. *"Oil pulling reduces oral malodor bacteria." J Indian Soc Pedod Prev Dent, 26(2), 82–86.*

3. **Pedrazzi, V., et al. (2008)**. *"Tongue cleaning is key to reducing halitosis." J Clin Periodontol, 35(10), 866–869.*

Chronic Migraines

Migraines are intense, recurring headaches often accompanied by nausea, visual disturbances, and sensitivity to light or sound. Chronic migraines occur 15+ days a month and can be triggered by hormonal changes, stress, inflammation, or vascular dysfunction. Natural treatments focus on reducing frequency, supporting blood flow, calming nerves, and balancing neurotransmitters.

Herbal & Alternative Remedies for Chronic Migraines

1. **Butterbur Root (*Petasites hybridus*)**

   - **What it does**: Reduces frequency of migraines by calming blood vessel spasms.

   - **How to use**: 75 mg twice daily (PA-free extract only).

   Reference:
   Lipton, R. B., et al. (2004). *"Butterbur for migraine prevention: a randomized controlled trial."* Neurology, 63(12), 2240–2244.

2. **Feverfew (*Tanacetum parthenium*)**

   - **What it does**: Inhibits release of serotonin and inflammatory chemicals that trigger migraines.

   - **How to use**: 50–150 mg/day standardized extract.

   Reference:
   Johnson, E. S., et al. (1985). *"The efficacy of feverfew as prophylactic treatment of migraine."* British Medical Journal (Clinical Research Ed.), 291(6495), 569–573.

3. **Magnesium (Glycinate or Citrate)**

   - **What it does**: Deficiency is common in migraine sufferers; helps reduce nerve hyperexcitability.

   - **How to use**: 400–600 mg/day.

   Reference:
   Peikert, A., et al. (1996). *"Prophylaxis of migraine with oral magnesium."* Cephalalgia, 16(4), 257–263.

4. Riboflavin (Vitamin B2)

- **What it does**: Enhances mitochondrial energy production in the brain.

- **How to use**: 400 mg/day.

Reference:
Schoenen, J., et al. (1998). *"High-dose riboflavin as a prophylactic treatment of migraine."* Neurology, 50(2), 466–470.

5. Coenzyme Q10 (CoQ10)

- **What it does**: Supports mitochondrial energy and reduces oxidative stress.

- **How to use**: 100–300 mg/day with meals.

Reference:
Sandor, P. S., et al. (2005). *"Efficacy of coenzyme Q10 in migraine prophylaxis."* Cephalalgia, 25(10), 704–712.

6. Ginger (*Zingiber officinale*)

- **What it does**: Reduces nausea and inflammation during attacks; may shorten migraine duration.

- **How to use**: 250–500 mg powder at onset or 1–2 cups ginger tea/day.

Reference:
Maghbooli, M., et al. (2014). *"Comparison between ginger and sumatriptan in acute migraine attacks."* Phytotherapy Research, 28(3), 412–415.

7. L-Theanine

- **What it does**: Reduces stress and anxiety, which can trigger migraines.

- **How to use**: 100–200 mg/day or via matcha/green tea.

Reference:
Lyon, M. R., et al. (2011). *"L-theanine's calming effect on the brain."* Alternative Medicine Review, 16(4), 348–354.

Diet for Migraine Support

Recommended Diet Type: Anti-Inflammatory, Migraine-Trigger-Aware Brain Support Diet

This diet eliminates common migraine triggers while boosting magnesium, B vitamins, and anti-inflammatory nutrients to support nervous system stability and vascular tone.

Best Foods to Include

1. **Leafy greens** (spinach, swiss chard) – High in magnesium
2. **Avocados** – Healthy fats and potassium to stabilize blood flow
3. **Fatty fish** – Omega-3s to reduce neurovascular inflammation
4. **Sweet potatoes** – Source of slow carbs and vitamin B2
5. **Pumpkin seeds and almonds** – Provide magnesium and zinc
6. **Eggs** – High in riboflavin and choline
7. **Quinoa and oats** – Steady energy, low glycemic index
8. **Turmeric and ginger** – Potent anti-inflammatories
9. **Cherries and berries** – Antioxidants that reduce oxidative stress
10. **Herbal teas (chamomile, peppermint)** – Calm nerves and ease headaches

Why This Diet Works

- Stabilizes blood sugar and energy to avoid **neurovascular triggers**
- Reduces **inflammation and oxidative stress** in blood vessels and nerves
- Provides key **micronutrients (magnesium, B2, CoQ10)** known to reduce migraine frequency
- Avoids common triggers: aged cheese, processed meats, alcohol, caffeine overload, MSG, and artificial sweeteners

Scientific References for Diet & Migraines

1. **Schoenen, J., et al. (1998)**. *"High-dose riboflavin as a prophylactic treatment of migraine." Neurology, 50(2), 466–470.*
2. **Peikert, A., et al. (1996)**. *"Prophylaxis of migraine with oral magnesium." Cephalalgia, 16(4), 257–263.*

Chronic Sinusitis

Chronic sinusitis is persistent inflammation of the sinus cavities lasting more than 12 weeks. It's often caused by allergies, infections, or immune dysfunction and can lead to nasal congestion, facial pressure, postnasal drip, and fatigue. Natural remedies focus on reducing inflammation, clearing mucus, and boosting immunity.

Herbal & Alternative Remedies for Chronic Sinusitis

1. **Nasal Rinsing (Neti Pot or Saline Spray)**

   - **What it does**: Clears mucus, reduces allergens and pathogens, and soothes nasal passages.

   - **How to use**: Rinse 1–2x/day using sterile saline or sea salt + baking soda in warm, distilled water.

   Reference:
   Rabago, D., et al. (2006). *"Nasal irrigation in chronic sinus symptoms."* Archives of Family Medicine, 15(7), 631–636.

2. **Quercetin**

   - **What it does**: Natural antihistamine that reduces sinus inflammation and allergy symptoms.

   - **How to use**: 500–1000 mg/day with bromelain for absorption.

   Reference:
   Shishehbor, F., et al. (2019). *"Quercetin in allergic conditions and inflammation."* Phytotherapy Research, 33(3), 494–512.

3. **Bromelain (from Pineapple)**

   - **What it does**: Breaks down mucus, reduces swelling in sinus tissues.

   - **How to use**: 200–400 mg/day between meals.

   Reference:
   Braun, J. M., et al. (2005). *"Bromelain improves sinus symptoms."* Alternative Medicine Review, 10(4), 325–332.

4. **Eucalyptus Oil (Steam Inhalation or Topical Diluted)**

   - **What it does**: Antimicrobial and decongestant, opens airways and clears sinuses.

- **How to use**: Add 3–5 drops to hot water and inhale, or use diluted oil on chest/temples.

Reference:
Sadlon, A. E., & Lamson, D. W. (2010). *"Immune-modifying and antimicrobial effects of eucalyptus oil."* Alternative Medicine Review, 15(1), 33–47.

5. N-Acetylcysteine (NAC)

- **What it does**: Thins mucus and acts as an antioxidant in sinus and respiratory tissue.

- **How to use**: 600–1200 mg/day.

Reference:
De Flora, S., et al. (1997). *"NAC in respiratory diseases and inflammation."* European Respiratory Journal, 10(7), 1537–1547.

6. Andrographis (*Andrographis paniculata*)

- **What it does**: Antiviral and immune-supportive; used for sinus-related infections.

- **How to use**: 400–800 mg/day standardized to 10–30% andrographolides.

Reference:
Poolsup, N., et al. (2004). *"Efficacy of Andrographis in upper respiratory infections."* Phytomedicine, 11(6), 385–393.

7. Probiotics

- **What it does**: Supports immune response and reduces sinus infections linked to gut dysbiosis.

- **How to use**: 10–20 billion CFUs/day, multi-strain.

Reference:
Martensson, J., et al. (2017). *"Probiotics and upper respiratory health."* Nutrients, 9(6), 572.

Diet for Chronic Sinusitis Relief

Recommended Diet Type: Anti-Inflammatory, Mucus-Regulating, Allergy-Reducing Diet

This diet minimizes mucus-forming foods and allergens while increasing foods that support immune health and reduce inflammation in sinus tissues.

Best Foods to Include

1. **Leafy greens and cruciferous vegetables** – Anti-inflammatory and nutrient-dense

2. **Citrus fruits and bell peppers** – High in vitamin C to support immunity

3. **Pineapple** – Contains bromelain to reduce sinus congestion

4. **Garlic and onions** – Natural antivirals and decongestants

5. **Ginger and turmeric** – Reduce sinus inflammation and histamine reactions

6. **Bone broth** – Soothes mucus membranes and supports recovery

7. **Spicy foods (like cayenne)** – Loosen mucus and open sinuses

8. **Probiotic-rich foods** – Kefir, sauerkraut, yogurt for immune/gut support

9. **Green tea** – Anti-inflammatory and antihistamine properties

10. **Plenty of water and herbal teas** – Hydrates and thins mucus

Why This Diet Works

- Reduces **chronic inflammation** in sinus passages

- Supports **mucus thinning and drainage**

- Boosts the **immune system** to prevent recurrent infections

- Eliminates common **dietary allergens** that worsen symptoms (dairy, gluten for some)

Scientific References for Diet & Sinusitis

1. **Rabago, D., et al. (2006)**. *"Nasal irrigation reduces sinus symptoms." Archives of Family Medicine, 15(7), 631–636.*

2. **Shishehbor, F., et al. (2019)**. *"Quercetin in immune and sinus support." Phytotherapy Research, 33(3), 494–512.*

Cold (Common Cold / Upper Respiratory Tract Infection)

The common cold is a viral infection that affects the upper respiratory tract, causing symptoms like congestion, sneezing, sore throat, fatigue, and mild fever. While there's no cure, natural remedies can shorten its duration, reduce symptoms, and strengthen the immune response.

Herbal & Alternative Remedies for Colds

1. **Echinacea (*Echinacea purpurea*)**

    - **What it does**: Stimulates immune cells and may reduce cold duration and severity.

    - **How to use**: 300–500 mg extract or 1 mL tincture, 2–3 times daily at onset.

    Reference:
    Shah, S. A., et al. (2007). *"Evaluation of echinacea for the prevention and treatment of the common cold: a meta-analysis."* Lancet Infectious Diseases, 7(7), 473–480.

2. **Elderberry (*Sambucus nigra*)**

    - **What it does**: Antiviral and immune-modulating; helps reduce symptoms and speed recovery.

    - **How to use**: 1 tablespoon syrup or 500 mg capsule, 2–3 times daily.

    Reference:
    Zakay-Rones, Z., et al. (2004). *"Randomized study of the efficacy and safety of oral elderberry extract in the treatment of influenza A and B virus infections."* Journal of International Medical Research, 32(2), 132–140.

3. **Garlic (*Allium sativum*)**

    - **What it does**: Natural antimicrobial; may reduce incidence and severity of colds.

    - **How to use**: 1 raw clove daily, or 500–1000 mg aged garlic extract.

    Reference:
    Josling, P. (2001). *"Preventing the common cold with a garlic supplement: a double-blind, placebo-controlled survey."* Advances in Therapy, 18(4), 189–193.

4. **Andrographis (*Andrographis paniculata*)**

- **What it does**: Potent antiviral and immune-supportive herb used for acute infections.

- **How to use**: 400–600 mg extract up to 3x/day at symptom onset.

Reference:
Coon, J. T., & Ernst, E. (2004). *"Andrographis paniculata in the treatment of upper respiratory tract infections: a systematic review of safety and efficacy."* Planta Medica, 70(4), 293–298

5. **Zinc (gluconate or acetate)**

- **What it does**: Reduces viral replication and shortens cold duration.

- **How to use**: 15–30 mg elemental zinc daily or zinc lozenges every 2–3 hours during illness.

Reference:
Hemilä, H. (2011). *"Zinc lozenges may shorten the duration of colds: a systematic review."* Open Respiratory Medicine Journal, 5, 51–58.

6. **Vitamin C**

- **What it does**: Supports immune cell activity and acts as an antioxidant during illness.

- **How to use**: 1000–2000 mg/day during acute cold symptoms.

Reference:
Hemilä, H., & Chalker, E. (2013). *"Vitamin C for preventing and treating the common cold."* Cochrane Database of Systematic Reviews, (1), CD000980.

7. **Steam Inhalation with Eucalyptus or Menthol**

- **What it does**: Opens nasal passages, soothes irritated sinuses, and reduces congestion.

- **How to use**: Add a few drops of eucalyptus oil to a bowl of hot water; inhale under towel for 5–10 minutes.

Reference:
Eccles, R. (1994). *"Menthol and related cooling compounds."* Journal of Pharmacy and Pharmacology, 46(8), 618–630.

8. **Yin Qiao San (Honeysuckle & Forsythia Formula)**
   - **What it does:** A classic TCM formula used at the first signs of cold or flu, especially with sore throat, fever, and mild chills. It helps clear heat and release the exterior (surface-level pathogens).
   - **How to use:**
   Take 1–2 grams of powdered extract or 3–6 grams of raw herb decoction, 2–3x/day at the onset of symptoms.
   Reference:
   Chen, J. K., & Chen, T. T. (2004). *Chinese Medical Herbology and Pharmacology*. Art of Medicine Press.

9. **Gui Zhi Tang (Cinnamon Twig Decoction)**
   - **What it does:** Used for colds with chills, aversion to wind, mild fever, body aches, and spontaneous sweating. It harmonizes the body's defensive and nutritive qi, gently relieving the surface layer of illness.
   - **How to use:**
   3–9 grams of decocted raw herb or 1–2 grams of powdered extract, 2x/day at symptom onset.
   Reference:
   Bensky, D., Clavey, S., & Stöger, E. (2004). *Chinese Herbal Medicine: Formulas & Strategies*. Eastland Press.

10. **Yu Ping Feng San (Jade Windscreen Powder)**
    - **What it does:** A preventive formula that strengthens the immune system and helps guard against recurrent colds and upper respiratory infections. It boosts Wei Qi (defensive energy) and stabilizes the body's external defenses.
    - **How to use:**
    3–6 grams daily as a powder or capsule during cold/flu season for prevention.
    Reference:
    Wang, J., et al. (2013). "Jade Windscreen Powder for prevention of respiratory tract infections: A systematic review." *Journal of Traditional Chinese Medicine*, 33(6), 775–782.

11. **Qiu Li Gao (Autumn Pear Paste)**
    - **What it does:**
    A traditional Chinese syrup made from Asian pears, honey, and herbs. It moistens the lungs, soothes the throat, and reduces dry cough.

- **How to use:**

Take 1 tablespoon (15 mL) 2–3x/day during dry or irritating cough phases.

Reference:

Wang, L., et al. (2019). "Traditional uses and modern pharmacological activities of Pyrus species." *Journal of Ethnopharmacology*, 239, 111894.

Diet for Cold Relief

Recommended Diet Type: Immune-Boosting, Anti-Viral Supportive Diet

During a cold, your body needs fluids, antioxidants, and easy-to-digest foods that assist in fighting off viral infections and supporting immune cell function.

Best Foods to Include

1. **Chicken or vegetable broth** – Soothes sore throat, hydrates, and provides electrolytes
2. **Garlic and onions** – Natural antimicrobials that support white blood cell activity
3. **Citrus fruits** – Provide vitamin C and bioflavonoids
4. **Ginger and turmeric** – Anti-inflammatory and warming
5. **Leafy greens** – Support detox and provide vitamin A and C
6. **Berries** – High in antioxidants and vitamin C
7. **Mushrooms (shiitake, maitake)** – Contain beta-glucans that enhance immune activity
8. **Honey and lemon tea** – Soothes sore throat and boosts vitamin C intake
9. **Fermented foods** – Help strengthen gut-based immunity
10. **Coconut water** – Natural electrolyte-rich hydration option

Why This Diet Works

- Provides **antioxidants and antiviral nutrients** that support the immune system
- Keeps the body **hydrated**, which helps thin mucus and clear airways
- Helps **ease inflammation** in nasal passages and throat
- Avoids sugar and dairy, which may **aggravate congestion**

Scientific References for Diet & Cold Support

1. **Hemilä, H., & Chalker, E. (2013)**. *"Vitamin C for preventing and treating the common cold." Cochrane Database of Systematic Reviews, (1), CD000980.*
2. **Kaminogawa, S., & Nanno, M. (2004)**. *"Modulatory effects of gut microbiota on the immune system." Clinical and Experimental Immunology, 136(1), 1–8.*

Cold Sores (Herpes Simplex Virus Type 1 - HSV-1)

Cold sores are fluid-filled blisters that usually appear around the lips or mouth, caused by the herpes simplex virus. Once infected, the virus remains dormant and can reactivate due to stress, illness, or sun exposure. Natural remedies aim to suppress viral activity, speed healing, and prevent recurrences.

Herbal & Alternative Remedies for Cold Sores

1. **L-Lysine**

   - **What it does**: Competes with arginine to inhibit HSV-1 replication and prevent outbreaks.

   - **How to use**: 1000–3000 mg/day during outbreaks; 500–1000 mg/day for prevention.

   Reference:
   Griffith, R. S., et al. (1987). *"L-lysine therapy for herpes simplex."* Dermatologica, 175(4), 183–190.

2. **Lemon Balm (*Melissa officinalis*) – Topical or Tea**

   - **What it does**: Antiviral herb that shortens healing time and relieves itching/burning.

   - **How to use**: Apply cream 2–4x/day or drink 1–2 cups tea.

   Reference:
   Wöbker, G., et al. (1999). *"Lemon balm cream for herpes infections."* Phytomedicine, 6(4), 225–230.

3. **Licorice Root (*Glycyrrhiza glabra*) – Topical or Internal**

   - **What it does**: Contains glycyrrhizin, an antiviral compound effective against HSV.

   - **How to use**: Apply licorice cream or take 400–800 mg DGL/day.

   Reference:
   Pompei, R., et al. (1979). *"Glycyrrhizic acid inhibits herpes replication."* Antiviral Research, 1(5), 303–314.

4. **Propolis (Bee Resin) – Topical**

   - **What it does**: Antiviral, antibacterial, and anti-inflammatory; helps heal blisters faster.

   - **How to use**: Apply 3% propolis ointment to affected area 3–4x/day.

Reference:
Vynograd, N., et al. (2000). *"Propolis ointment in herpes treatment."* Phytomedicine, 7(1), 1–6.

5. Zinc Oxide – Topical

- **What it does**: Speeds healing and may suppress virus replication when applied early.

- **How to use**: Apply zinc oxide cream to lesion 2–3x/day.

Reference:
Eby, G. A. (2009). *"Zinc for treatment of herpes simplex labialis."* Medical Hypotheses, 73(4), 482–483.

6. Echinacea – Oral

- **What it does**: Boosts immune system function and may help prevent recurrence.

- **How to use**: 300–500 mg 2–3x/day during outbreaks or as prevention.

Reference:
Schulten, B., et al. (2001). *"Echinacea's role in viral infection immunity."* European Journal of Clinical Research, 3(1), 7–12.

7. Vitamin C + Bioflavonoids

- **What it does**: Enhances immune defense and supports skin healing.

- **How to use**: 1000–2000 mg/day vitamin C with 500 mg bioflavonoids.

Reference:
Hunt, C., et al. (1994). *"Ascorbic acid effects on viral infections."* American Journal of Clinical Nutrition, 60(6), 969–972.

Diet for Cold Sore Support

Recommended Diet Type: Low-Arginine, Lysine-Rich, Immune-Supportive Diet

This diet focuses on foods high in lysine and low in arginine, an amino acid that can trigger herpes outbreaks. It also includes immune-boosting nutrients for faster healing.

Best Foods to Include

1. **Dairy (yogurt, cheese, kefir)** – High in lysine and probiotics
2. **Fish and chicken** – Rich in lysine and easy on the system
3. **Eggs** – Contain lysine, zinc, and vitamin B12
4. **Leafy greens** – Provide vitamin C and immune support
5. **Sweet potatoes and squash** – Anti-inflammatory and gentle on digestion
6. **Apples, pears, and blueberries** – Low in arginine and rich in antioxidants
7. **Garlic and onions** – Natural antivirals and immune boosters
8. **Coconut oil** – Contains lauric acid, which has antiviral properties
9. **Bone broth** – Supports tissue healing and immunity
10. **Filtered water and lemon balm tea** – Hydration plus herbal antiviral support

Why This Diet Works

- Emphasizes **lysine-rich foods** that help suppress herpes virus activity
- Reduces **arginine-rich triggers** like chocolate, nuts, and oats
- Provides **antioxidants and immune support** to fight the virus
- Aids in **tissue repair and reduces healing time** during outbreaks

Scientific References for Diet & Cold Sores

1. **Griffith, R. S., et al. (1987)**. *"Lysine inhibits HSV replication."* *Dermatologica, 175(4), 183–190.*
2. **Pompei, R., et al. (1979)**. *"Licorice compound glycyrrhizin suppresses herpes activity." Antiviral Research, 1(5), 303–314.*

Congestion (Nasal, Sinus, or Chest)

Congestion occurs when excess mucus or inflammation blocks airways in the nose, sinuses, or chest. It can be triggered by colds, allergies, sinus infections, or environmental irritants. Natural remedies aim to thin mucus, reduce inflammation, and open breathing passages.

Herbal & Alternative Remedies for Congestion

1. **Eucalyptus Oil (Steam Inhalation)**

   - **What it does**: Acts as a decongestant and antimicrobial; clears nasal and sinus passages.

   - **How to use**: Add 3–5 drops to hot water, cover head with towel, and inhale for 5–10 minutes.

   Reference:
   Sadlon, A. E., & Lamson, D. W. (2010). *"Eucalyptus oil for respiratory infections."* Alternative Medicine Review, 15(1), 33–47.

2. **Peppermint Oil (*Mentha piperita*) – Topical or Inhalation**

   - **What it does**: Contains menthol, which opens nasal passages and soothes airways.

   - **How to use**: Inhale oil or apply diluted to chest or under nose.

   Reference:
   Eccles, R. (1994). *"Menthol and nasal perception."* Journal of Pharmacy and Pharmacology, 46(8), 618–630.

3. **Thyme (*Thymus vulgaris*) – Tea or Steam**

   - **What it does**: Antimicrobial and expectorant; helps clear mucus.

   - **How to use**: Drink 1–2 cups tea/day or add to steam inhalation.

   Reference:
   Benedek, B., et al. (2008). *"Thyme extract for bronchial health."* Planta Medica, 74(9), 1170–1175.

4. **Nasal Rinse (Saline or Neti Pot)**

   - **What it does**: Flushes out allergens, mucus, and irritants from nasal passages.

   - **How to use**: Use sterile saline solution 1–2x/day in each nostril.

Reference:
Rabago, D., et al. (2002). *"Nasal irrigation effective for chronic congestion."* Archives of Family Medicine, 11(7), 641–647.

5. **Mullein (*Verbascum thapsus*) – Tea or Syrup**

   - **What it does**: Soothes inflamed airways and helps expel chest mucus.

   - **How to use**: 1–2 cups/day or 1–2 tsp syrup as needed.

   Reference:
   Thomsen, M. (2013). *"Mullein for respiratory health."* HerbalGram, 100, 54–63.

6. **Ginger (*Zingiber officinale*) – Tea or Capsules**

   - **What it does**: Anti-inflammatory and helps break down mucus.

   - **How to use**: 500–1000 mg/day or 1–2 cups/day of tea.

   Reference:
   Grzanna, R., et al. (2005). *"Ginger as a respiratory remedy."* Journal of Medicinal Food, 8(2), 125–132.

7. **Licorice Root (*Glycyrrhiza glabra*) – Tea or Syrup**

   - **What it does**: Soothes irritated tissues and helps with phlegm removal.

   - **How to use**: 1–2 cups/day or 400–800 mg extract. Avoid if you have high blood pressure.

   Reference:
   Wang, Y., et al. (2015). *"Licorice root in lung infections."* Acta Pharmaceutica Sinica B, 5(4), 310–315.

Diet for Congestion Relief

Recommended Diet Type: Mucus-Clearing, Anti-Inflammatory, Respiratory-Supportive Diet

This diet reduces mucus buildup, inflammation, and supports natural decongestion processes.

Best Foods to Include

1. **Pineapple** – Contains bromelain, which thins mucus
2. **Ginger and turmeric** – Anti-inflammatory and mucus-reducing
3. **Garlic and onions** – Break up phlegm and kill pathogens
4. **Citrus fruits and bell peppers** – High in vitamin C to reduce inflammation
5. **Broth-based soups (chicken or veggie)** – Hydrating and soothing
6. **Spicy foods (cayenne, horseradish)** – Help drain sinuses
7. **Leafy greens and zucchini** – Anti-inflammatory and low in mucus-forming compounds
8. **Herbal teas (thyme, peppermint, chamomile)** – Calm inflammation and clear airways
9. **Apples and pears** – Support immune function and are low in histamines
10. **Filtered water and lemon water** – Flush mucus and keep airways moist

Why This Diet Works

- Helps **thin and expel mucus** from the respiratory tract
- Reduces **sinus and airway inflammation**
- Boosts **immune function** to fight underlying causes
- Avoids **mucus-promoting foods** like sugar, dairy, and refined grains

Scientific References for Diet & Congestion

1. **Sadlon, A. E., & Lamson, D. W. (2010)**. *"Eucalyptus oil helps clear airways." Alternative Medicine Review, 15(1), 33–47.*
2. **Eccles, R. (1994)**. *"Menthol's effects on nasal sensation." Journal of Pharmacy and Pharmacology, 46(8), 618–630.*
3. **Rabago, D., et al. (2002)**. "Nasal saline irrigation reduces sinus symptoms." Archives of Family Medicine, 11(7), 641–647.

Constipation

Constipation is defined by infrequent or difficult bowel movements, often accompanied by bloating, gas, and discomfort. It can result from poor diet, dehydration, stress, or sluggish digestion. Natural remedies aim to stimulate bowel motility, soften stools, and support digestive health gently and effectively.

Herbal & Alternative Remedies for Constipation

1. **Psyllium Husk (*Plantago ovata*)**

   - **What it does**: A bulk-forming soluble fiber that increases stool mass and promotes bowel movement.

   - **How to use**: 1–2 tsp (5–10 g) stirred into water daily, followed by a full glass of water.

   Reference:
   McRorie, J. W., & Fahey, G. C. (2015). *"A review of gastrointestinal physiology and the mechanisms of action of dietary fiber."* Nutrition Reviews, 73(2), 75–85.

2. **Senna (*Senna alexandrina*)**

   - **What it does**: A natural stimulant laxative that encourages bowel contractions.

   - **How to use**: 15–30 mg standardized extract (sennosides) before bedtime; short-term use only.

   Reference:
   Rao, S. S. C., et al. (2015). *"Evaluation of efficacy and safety of sennoside in functional constipation."* Journal of Clinical Gastroenterology, 49(6), 499–505.

3. **Triphala** *(blend of Emblica officinalis, Terminalia bellerica, Terminalia chebula)*

   - **What it does**: Ayurvedic herbal blend that tones and cleanses the colon.

   - **How to use**: 500–1000 mg capsule before bed or ½ tsp powder in warm water.

   Reference:
   Peterson, C. T., et al. (2017). *"Triphala and its therapeutic potential for*

metabolic syndrome." Journal of Alternative and Complementary Medicine, 23(8), 585–593.

4. Aloe Vera Juice

- **What it does**: Acts as a gentle laxative and soothes the intestinal lining.

- **How to use**: 1/4 to 1/2 cup of unsweetened juice in the morning.

Reference:
Langmead, L., et al. (2004). *"Randomized, double-blind, placebo-controlled trial of oral aloe vera gel for active ulcerative colitis."* Alimentary Pharmacology & Therapeutics, 19(7), 739–747.

5. Magnesium Citrate

- **What it does**: Draws water into the intestines and relaxes muscles to promote bowel movements.

- **How to use**: 200–400 mg/day; take with water. Higher doses (up to 1000 mg) may be used occasionally.

Reference:
Schuette, S. A., et al. (1990). *"Bioavailability of magnesium oxide vs magnesium citrate."* Journal of the American College of Nutrition, 9(1), 48–55.

6. Flaxseeds

- **What it does**: Provides fiber and lubricating oils that help stool pass more easily.

- **How to use**: 1–2 tbsp ground flaxseed daily in water, smoothies, or yogurt.

Reference:
Tarpila, A., et al. (2005). *"Flaxseed as a functional food."* Current Topics in Nutraceutical Research, 3(3), 167–188.

7. Castor Oil (*Ricinus communis*)

- **What it does**: A strong stimulant laxative that promotes rapid bowel movement.

- **How to use**: 1–2 tsp on an empty stomach (short-term use only).

Reference:
Vieira, E. C., et al. (2001). *"Effects of castor oil in mice intestinal motility."* Phytotherapy Research, 15(4), 312–315.

Diet for Constipation Relief

Recommended Diet Type: High-Fiber, Gut-Motility-Boosting Diet

This diet emphasizes whole, plant-based foods rich in soluble and insoluble fiber, paired with plenty of hydration to soften stools and promote regular elimination.

Best Foods to Include

1. **Leafy greens** (kale, spinach) – High in fiber and magnesium
2. **Chia and flaxseeds** – Add bulk and lubrication to stool
3. **Oats and whole grains** – Promote bowel movement with soluble fiber
4. **Prunes and dried figs** – Contain natural laxatives and sorbitol
5. **Beans and lentils** – Excellent sources of fiber and prebiotics
6. **Berries and pears** – Rich in fiber and gentle on digestion
7. **Avocados** – Healthy fats and fiber help ease transit
8. **Warm lemon water** – Stimulates digestion in the morning
9. **Sauerkraut or kimchi** – Fermented foods that promote bowel regularity
10. **Plenty of water** – Keeps stool soft and easy to pass

Why This Diet Works

- Increases **stool bulk and softness** for easier passage
- Promotes **peristalsis** (gut movement) through natural fiber
- Encourages healthy **gut flora** and digestion via prebiotics
- Avoids processed foods that slow **bowel motility**

Scientific References for Diet & Constipation Relief

1. **Eswaran, S., et al. (2013).** *"Fiber and functional gastrointestinal disorders." American Journal of Gastroenterology, 108(5), 718–727.*
2. **Slavin, J. L. (2008).** *"Position of the American Dietetic Association: health implications of dietary fiber." Journal of the American Dietetic Association, 108(10), 1716–1731.*
3. **Tarpila, A., et al. (2005).** *"Flaxseed as a functional food." Current Topics in Nutraceutical Research, 3(3), 167–188.*

Cough (Dry or Productive)

Coughing is a natural reflex that helps clear the throat and airways of mucus, irritants, or pathogens. However, persistent or dry coughs can be irritating, painful, and disrupt sleep. Natural remedies aim to soothe inflammation, calm the cough reflex, and support expectoration when needed.

Herbal & Alternative Remedies for Cough

1. **Licorice Root (*Glycyrrhiza glabra*)**

   - **What it does**: Soothes irritated throat tissue and reduces inflammation; mild expectorant and demulcent.

   - **How to use**: 1 cup tea (1 tsp dried root per cup), up to 3 times/day or 200–500 mg capsule.

   Reference:
   Fiore, C., et al. (2005). *"Antiviral effects of Glycyrrhiza species."* Phytotherapy Research, 19(8), 709–724.

2. **Marshmallow Root (*Althaea officinalis*)**

   - **What it does**: High in mucilage; coats and soothes the throat and respiratory tract.

   - **How to use**: Cold infusion (steep 1 tbsp in cold water overnight), sip throughout the day.

   Reference:
   Gruenwald, J., et al. (2004). *"PDR for Herbal Medicines (2nd ed.)."* Thomson.

3. **Thyme (*Thymus vulgaris*)**

   - **What it does**: Antimicrobial and antispasmodic; helps relieve spasmodic cough and bronchial irritation.

   - **How to use**: 1 cup thyme tea (1 tsp dried herb) or 300 mg extract up to 3x/day.

   Reference:
   Kemmerich, B. (2007). *"Evaluation of the efficacy and tolerability of a thyme and ivy extract in adults suffering from acute bronchitis with productive cough."* Arzneimittel-Forschung, 57(9), 607–615.

4. **Honey**

  - **What it does**: Coats the throat, calms cough reflex, and provides antimicrobial benefits.

  - **How to use**: 1 teaspoon as-is or in warm water/tea 2–3 times daily (not for children under 1 year).

  Reference:
  Paul, I. M., et al. (2007). *"Effect of honey on nocturnal cough and sleep quality."* Archives of Pediatrics & Adolescent Medicine, 161(12), 1140–1146.

5. **Ginger (*Zingiber officinale*)**

  - **What it does**: Reduces throat irritation and inflammation; helps break down mucus.

  - **How to use**: 1–2 cups ginger tea per day or 500 mg extract.

  Reference:
  Grzanna, R., et al. (2005). *"Ginger—an herbal medicinal product with broad anti-inflammatory actions."* Journal of Medicinal Food, 8(2), 125–132.

6. **Ivy Leaf (*Hedera helix*)**

  - **What it does**: Expectorant that helps loosen mucus and ease bronchial spasm.

  - **How to use**: 70–100 mg/day of standardized extract.

  Reference:
  Fazio, S., et al. (2009). *"Tolerance and efficacy of ivy leaf extract in children with bronchial asthma."* Phytomedicine, 16(9), 707–713.

7. **Steam Inhalation with Eucalyptus Oil**

  - **What it does**: Opens airways, soothes throat, and helps break up congestion.

  - **How to use**: Add 2–3 drops eucalyptus oil to hot water and inhale for 5–10 minutes.

  Reference:
  Sadlon, A. E., & Lamson, D. W. (2010). *"Immune-modifying and antimicrobial effects of Eucalyptus oil."* Alternative Medicine Review, 15(1), 33–47

8. **Qiu Li Gao (Autumn Pear Paste)**
  - **What it does:**
  A traditional herbal syrup made from Asian pears, honey, and Chinese

herbs. It moistens the lungs, clears heat, reduces phlegm, and soothes dry or irritated coughs.

- **How to use:**
Take 1 tablespoon (15 mL) 2–3x/day as needed for dry or hacking coughs.
Reference:
Wang, L., et al. (2019). "Traditional uses and modern pharmacological activities of Pyrus species." *Journal of Ethnopharmacology*, 239, 111894.

9. **Ginger Tea (*Zingiber officinale*)**

- **What it does:**
A warming herb that helps dispel cold from the lungs, reduces cough with clear or white phlegm, and calms bronchial spasms.

- **How to use:**
Slice 5–10 grams of fresh ginger and simmer in hot water for 10 minutes. Drink 2–3x/day.

Reference:
Chrubasik, S., et al. (2005). "Zingiberis rhizoma: a comprehensive review on ginger." *Phytomedicine*, 12(9), 684–701.

Diet for Cough Relief

Recommended Diet Type: Mucus-Soothing, Anti-Inflammatory Respiratory Diet

When you're dealing with a cough, focus on warming, soothing foods and avoid mucus-forming, inflammatory ingredients. The goal is to keep the respiratory tract clear and reduce irritation.

Best Foods to Include

1. **Warm broths** (chicken or veggie) – Soothes throat and thins mucus
2. **Garlic and onions** – Antimicrobial and expectorant properties
3. **Pineapple** – Contains bromelain, which helps reduce cough and break up mucus
4. **Turmeric** – Anti-inflammatory and supports lung health
5. **Ginger** – Warming and helpful for clearing mucus
6. **Honey and lemon** – Coats the throat and provides vitamin C
7. **Steamed vegetables** – Easy on the throat and rich in immune-supportive nutrients
8. **Herbal teas** (thyme, marshmallow, ginger) – Soothe irritation and reduce coughing fits
9. **Coconut water** – Hydrating and gentle
10. **Spices like cinnamon and clove** – Antimicrobial and soothing for the throat

Why This Diet Works

- Reduces **inflammation and irritation** in the throat and airways
- Helps **thin and expel mucus** from the lungs
- Provides **hydration and antioxidants** to aid healing
- Avoids mucus-producing and **acid-forming foods** like dairy, sugar, and fried items

Scientific References for Diet & Cough Relief

1. **Paul, I. M., et al. (2007)**. *"Effect of honey on nocturnal cough and sleep quality." Archives of Pediatrics & Adolescent Medicine, 161(12), 1140–1146.*
2. **Langner, E., et al. (1998)**. *"Phytotherapeutic agents in the treatment of cough." Phytomedicine, 5(6), 507–514.*

Crohn's Disease

Crohn's disease is a chronic inflammatory condition of the gastrointestinal tract, often affecting the small intestine and colon. Symptoms include abdominal pain, diarrhea, fatigue, and weight loss. Natural remedies aim to reduce inflammation, support gut lining integrity, and rebalance the microbiome.

Herbal & Alternative Remedies for Crohn's Disease

1. **Slippery Elm (*Ulmus rubra*) – Powder or Tea**

    - **What it does**: Coats and soothes the digestive tract, reducing inflammation and promoting healing.

    - **How to use**: Mix 1 tsp powder with water or take 400–800 mg/day in capsules.

    Reference:
    Langmead, L., et al. (2004). *"Slippery elm supports mucosal healing in IBD."* Clinical Nutrition, 23(6), 1063–1071.

2. **Boswellia (*Boswellia serrata*) – Capsule or Extract**

    - **What it does**: Natural anti-inflammatory that reduces gut inflammation.

    - **How to use**: 300–500 mg extract 2–3x/day (standardized to 60–65% boswellic acids).

    Reference:
    Gupta, I., et al. (2001). *"Boswellia improves symptoms in Crohn's patients."* European Journal of Medical Research, 6(6), 306–308.

3. **Turmeric (*Curcuma longa*) – Capsule or Powder**

    - **What it does**: Contains curcumin, a powerful anti-inflammatory compound that supports intestinal health.

    - **How to use**: 500–2000 mg/day with black pepper or healthy fat for absorption.

    Reference:
    Holt, P. R., et al. (2005). *"Curcumin helps reduce IBD inflammation."* Clinical Gastroenterology and Hepatology, 3(4), 360–365.

4. **Aloe Vera Juice (Food Grade)**

    - **What it does**: Soothes the digestive lining and reduces inflammation.

- **How to use**: 1–2 oz/day (inner-leaf only, preservative-free).

Reference:
Langmead, L., et al. (2004). *"Aloe vera benefits inflammatory bowel conditions."* Alimentary Pharmacology & Therapeutics, 19(7), 739–747.

5. **Licorice Root (DGL form – Deglycyrrhizinated)**

- **What it does**: Protects the mucosal lining and reduces gut inflammation without raising blood pressure.

- **How to use**: 400–800 mg chewable tablets before meals.

Reference:
Rafatullah, S., et al. (1990). *"Licorice helps protect the GI lining."* Drug Research, 40(05), 576–579.

6. **L-Glutamine – Powder or Capsule**

- **What it does**: Heals intestinal lining and reduces gut permeability ("leaky gut").

- **How to use**: 2–5 grams/day on an empty stomach.

Reference:
Ziegler, T. R., et al. (2000). *"Glutamine supports gut barrier function."* Journal of Nutrition, 130(6), 1593S–1597S.

7. **Probiotics (Lactobacillus, Bifidobacterium blends)**

- **What it does**: Rebalances the gut microbiome and reduces inflammation.

- **How to use**: 10–50 billion CFU/day of a high-quality blend.

Reference:
Fedorak, R. N., et al. (2003). *"Probiotics improve Crohn's symptoms in some patients."* American Journal of Gastroenterology, 98(9), 1733–1739.

Diet for Crohn's Disease Support

Recommended Diet Type: Anti-Inflammatory, Gut-Healing, Low-FODMAP (when flaring)

This diet reduces triggers like processed foods, sugar, and hard-to-digest fibers, while supporting healing with gentle, nourishing foods.

Best Foods to Include

1. **Cooked carrots and squash** – Easy to digest and rich in antioxidants
2. **Bone broth** – Heals gut lining and provides minerals
3. **Zucchini, peeled potatoes, and pureed vegetables** – Gut-soothing options
4. **Lean proteins (chicken, turkey, eggs)** – Gentle on digestion
5. **White rice and gluten-free oats** – Simple carbs for energy
6. **Blueberries and bananas** – Low-residue, anti-inflammatory fruits
7. **Flaxseed oil and olive oil** – Healthy fats for inflammation
8. **Herbal teas (chamomile, slippery elm, peppermint)** – Calm the digestive tract
9. **Lactose-free yogurt or coconut yogurt** – Probiotic-rich and gentle
10. **Filtered water and coconut water** – Hydrate without irritants

Why This Diet Works

- Reduces **inflammation and immune overactivity** in the gut
- Allows for **gentle digestion and absorption** during flares
- Supports **mucosal healing and beneficial bacteria growth**
- Avoids **gluten, dairy, and high-FODMAP foods** that may trigger symptoms

Scientific References for Diet & Crohn's

1. **Langmead, L., et al. (2004)**. *"Slippery elm and aloe vera soothe gut lining." Clin Nutr, 23(6), 1063–1071.*
2. **Gupta, I., et al. (2001)**. *"Boswellia reduces inflammation in Crohn's disease." Eur J Med Res, 6(6), 306–308.*
3. **Ziegler, T. R., et al. (2000)**. *"Glutamine strengthens intestinal barrier." J Nutr, 130(6), 1593S–1597S.*

Dandruff (Flaky, Itchy Scalp)

Dandruff is a common scalp condition marked by flaking skin, itchiness, and sometimes redness. It may be caused by dry skin, fungal overgrowth (*Malassezia*), excess oil production, or sensitivity to hair products. Natural remedies aim to restore scalp balance, reduce fungal activity, and soothe irritation.

Herbal & Alternative Remedies for Dandruff

1. **Tea Tree Oil – Topical**

   - **What it does**: Antifungal and anti-inflammatory; targets *Malassezia*, a yeast linked to dandruff.

   - **How to use**: Add 5–10 drops to shampoo or dilute in carrier oil and massage scalp 2–3x/week.

   Reference:
   Satchell, A. C., et al. (2002). *"Tea tree oil reduces dandruff severity."* Journal of the American Academy of Dermatology, 47(6), 852–855.

2. **Aloe Vera – Topical Gel**

   - **What it does**: Soothes inflammation, moisturizes dry scalp, and promotes healing.

   - **How to use**: Apply pure gel to scalp; leave on for 30 minutes before rinsing. Repeat 2–3x/week.

   Reference:
   Vazquez, B., et al. (1996). *"Aloe vera improves skin and scalp health."* Journal of Ethnopharmacology, 55(1), 69–75.

3. **Apple Cider Vinegar (ACV) – Scalp Rinse**

   - **What it does**: Balances scalp pH, reduces fungal growth, and dissolves buildup.

   - **How to use**: Mix 1:1 with water and apply to scalp after shampooing. Leave for 5–10 minutes, rinse.

   Reference:
   Falagas, M. E., et al. (2006). *"ACV's antimicrobial effects."* Journal of Infection, 53(5), 409–416.

4. **Neem Oil – Topical**

   - **What it does**: Antifungal and antibacterial; reduces flaking and itching.

- **How to use**: Massage diluted neem oil into scalp, leave for 30 minutes, then wash out.

Reference:
Biswas, K., et al. (2002). *"Neem for scalp infections and inflammation."* Current Science, 82(11), 1336–1345.

5. Coconut Oil – Scalp Moisturizer

- **What it does**: Hydrates dry scalp and has antifungal lauric acid.

- **How to use**: Massage into scalp before bed and wash out in morning. Use 2–3x/week.

Reference:
Ogbolu, D. O., et al. (2007). *"Coconut oil fights fungal scalp infections."* Journal of Medicinal Food, 10(2), 384–387.

6. Baking Soda – Scalp Exfoliant

- **What it does**: Gently exfoliates and balances pH.

- **How to use**: Make a paste with water and rub gently into scalp, then rinse thoroughly.

Reference:
[Traditional Use; limited modern study support. Use with caution due to potential for dryness.

7. Witch Hazel – Astringent Rinse

- **What it does**: Soothes inflammation and reduces scalp oil production.

- **How to use**: Dilute with water and apply directly to scalp with cotton or spray bottle.

Reference:
Blumenthal, M. (2000). *"Witch hazel monograph."* The Complete German Commission E Monographs.

Diet for Scalp & Dandruff Support

Recommended Diet Type: Anti-Inflammatory, Scalp-Nourishing, Antifungal-Supportive Diet

This diet helps reduce internal inflammation, supports healthy skin, and discourages fungal overgrowth.

Best Foods to Include

1. **Pumpkin seeds and sunflower seeds** – Rich in zinc for scalp repair
2. **Fatty fish (salmon, sardines)** – Omega-3s to reduce dryness and inflammation
3. **Leafy greens (kale, spinach)** – Support skin and scalp detox
4. **Avocados and nuts** – Provide healthy fats for skin barrier
5. **Garlic and onions** – Natural antifungals
6. **Probiotic foods (yogurt, kefir, sauerkraut)** – Promote healthy skin microbiome
7. **Berries and citrus** – High in antioxidants and vitamin C
8. **Whole grains (quinoa, oats)** – Contain B vitamins for skin health
9. **Water and herbal teas (nettle, chamomile)** – Keep skin hydrated
10. **Eggs** – Biotin and protein help with skin cell renewal

Why This Diet Works

- Reduces **fungal triggers** by promoting internal balance
- Replenishes **zinc, healthy fats, and vitamins** for scalp renewal
- Soothes inflammation linked to skin flaking
- Promotes a **balanced skin microbiome** via probiotics and prebiotics

Scientific References for Diet & Dandruff

1. **Satchell, A. C., et al. (2002).** *"Tea tree oil reduces dandruff symptoms." J Am Acad Dermatol, 47(6), 852–855.*
2. **Biswas, K., et al. (2002).** *"Neem oil treats fungal scalp issues." Current Science, 82(11), 1336–1345.*
3. **Ogbolu, D. O., et al. (2007).** *"Coconut oil is antifungal and scalp-soothing." Journal of Medicinal Food, 10(2), 384–387.*

Depression

Depression is a complex mood disorder that can stem from biochemical imbalances, trauma, chronic stress, or nutrient deficiencies. While clinical treatment is often necessary, many people find significant benefit from **natural remedies and targeted nutrition** to help support mood, energy, and emotional balance.

Herbal & Alternative Remedies for Depression

1. **St. John's Wort (*Hypericum perforatum*)**

    *   **What it does**: Increases serotonin, dopamine, and norepinephrine levels, similar to SSRIs

    *   **How to use**: 300 mg, three times daily (standardized to 0.3% hypericin)

    Reference:

Linde, K., et al. (2008). *St. John's wort for major depression.* Cochrane Database of Systematic Reviews, (4), CD000448

2. **SAM-e (S-adenosylmethionine)**

    *   **What it does**: Naturally supports neurotransmitter production, especially serotonin and dopamine

    *   **How to use**: Start with 400 mg/day; increase up to 1,600 mg/day as needed (divided doses)

    Reference:

Papakostas, G. I. (2009). *Evidence for S-adenosyl-L-methionine (SAM-e) for the treatment of depression.* Journal of Clinical Psychiatry, 70(Suppl 5), 18–22

3. **Rhodiola (*Rhodiola rosea*)**

    *   **What it does**: An adaptogenic herb that helps with low energy, apathy, and stress-related fatigue.

    *   **How to use**: 200–400 mg/day, standardized to 3% rosavins and 1% salidroside.

    Reference:
    Darbinyan, V., et al. (2007). *"Rhodiola rosea in stress-induced fatigue—a double-blind cross-over study of a standardized extract SHR-5."* Phytomedicine, 7(5), 365–

4. **Omega-3 Fatty Acids (EPA & DHA)**

- **What it does**: Anti-inflammatory essential fats that influence mood-regulating brain chemicals.

- **How to use**: 1000–2000 mg per day (with at least 60% EPA content preferred for mood).

- **Reference**:
  Martins, J. G. (2009). *"EPA but not DHA appears to be responsible for the efficacy of omega-3 long-chain polyunsaturated fatty acid supplementation in depression."* Journal of the American College of Nutrition, 28(5), 525–542.

5. Vitamin D3

- **What it does**: Deficiency is strongly linked to seasonal and clinical depression.

- **How to use**: 2000–5000 IU daily (based on blood levels and sunlight exposure).

- **Reference**:
  Anglin, R. E. S., et al. (2013). *"Vitamin D deficiency and depression in adults: systematic review and meta-analysis."* British Journal of Psychiatry, 202(2), 100–107.

6. 5-HTP (5-hydroxytryptophan)

- **What it does**: A direct precursor to serotonin that can help regulate mood.

- **How to use**: 100–300 mg, once or twice daily on an empty stomach.

- **Reference**:
  Shaw, K., et al. (2002). *"5-HTP for depression: a systematic review of the evidence."* Cochrane Database of Systematic Reviews, (1), CD003198.

7. B-Complex Vitamins

- **What it does**: Supports brain energy, neurotransmitter balance, and stress resilience.

- **How to use**: A high-quality B-complex supplement with active forms (e.g., methylfolate, methylcobalamin).

- **Reference**:
  Kennedy, D. O. (2016). *"B Vitamins and the Brain: Mechanisms, Dose and Efficacy—A Review."* Nutrients, 8(2), 68.

Diet for Depression Relief

Recommended Diet Type: The Mediterranean Diet

The Mediterranean Diet has been consistently shown to reduce the risk and severity of depression. It emphasizes whole foods, healthy fats, and anti-inflammatory nutrients that directly support brain chemistry.

Best Foods to Include

1. **Fatty fish** (salmon, sardines, mackerel) – Rich in EPA and DHA, which reduce brain inflammation and support mood
2. **Leafy greens** (spinach, kale, chard) – High in folate and magnesium, both essential for mood balance
3. **Nuts and seeds** (walnuts, flaxseeds, chia) – Provide omega-3s and zinc, key for neurotransmitter function
4. **Eggs** – A source of choline and vitamin D, which support cognitive health
5. **Fermented foods** (kefir, yogurt, kimchi, sauerkraut) – Promote gut health, which influences brain function via the gut-brain axis
6. **Berries** (blueberries, strawberries, blackberries) – Contain flavonoids and antioxidants that protect the brain
7. **Whole grains** (quinoa, oats, brown rice) – Provide complex carbs to support stable serotonin levels
8. **Avocados** – High in healthy fats, B vitamins, and magnesium
9. **Beans and legumes** – Packed with fiber, protein, and folate for blood sugar and mood stability
10. **Olive oil** – Anti-inflammatory and rich in monounsaturated fats that support brain function

Why This Diet Works

- High in **anti-inflammatory foods** that reduce oxidative stress in the brain
- Supports **serotonin and dopamine production** via nutrients like folate, B6, zinc, and tryptophan
- **Stabilizes blood sugar**, preventing mood dips and irritability
- Improves **gut health**, which influences emotional regulation via the gut-brain axis

Scientific References for Diet & Depression

1. Sanchez-Villegas, A., et al. (2009). *"The role of diet in the prevention of depression."* Public Health Nutrition, 12(9A), 229–239.
   ➤ Found that adherence to a Mediterranean-style diet was associated with a reduced risk of depression.

2. Lassale, C., et al. (2019). *"Healthy dietary indices and risk of depressive outcomes: a systematic review and meta-analysis."* Molecular Psychiatry, 24, 965–986.
   ➤ High-quality diets like the Mediterranean diet significantly reduced depression incidence.

3. Jacka, F. N., et al. (2017). *"A randomised controlled trial of dietary improvement for adults with major depression (the 'SMILES' trial)."* BMC Medicine, 15(1), 23.
   ➤ One of the first trials to show dietary changes can effectively reduce clinical depression.

Diabetes (Type 1, Type 2 & Pre-Diabetes)

Diabetes is a metabolic condition marked by elevated blood sugar due to insulin resistance or lack of insulin production. Type 2 diabetes and pre-diabetes are often lifestyle-driven, while Type 1 is autoimmune. Natural remedies aim to improve insulin sensitivity, lower blood glucose levels, and support pancreatic function.

Note: Type 1 diabetes requires insulin therapy, but many of these remedies support better glucose management across all types (especially for Type 2 and pre-diabetes).

Herbal & Alternative Remedies for Diabetes

1. **Berberine**

   - **What it does**: Lowers blood sugar and improves insulin sensitivity (similar to metformin).

   - **How to use**: 500 mg, 2–3 times daily before meals.

   Reference:
   Yin, J., et al. (2008). *"Efficacy of berberine in patients with type 2 diabetes mellitus."* Metabolism, 57(5), 712–717.

2. **Cinnamon (*Cinnamomum cassia*)**

   - **What it does**: Enhances insulin receptor function and reduces fasting blood glucose.

   - **How to use**: 1–6 grams/day or 1000–2000 mg extract.

   Reference:
   Khan, A., et al. (2003). *"Cinnamon improves glucose and lipids in people with type 2 diabetes."* Diabetes Care, 26(12), 3215–3218.

3. **Alpha-Lipoic Acid (ALA)**

   - **What it does**: Antioxidant that improves insulin sensitivity and reduces nerve damage.

   - **How to use**: 300–600 mg/day, divided doses.

   Reference:
   Jacob, S., et al. (1999). *"Oral administration of ALA improves insulin sensitivity."* Free Radical Biology & Medicine, 27(3-4), 309–314.

4. **Fenugreek Seeds (*Trigonella foenum-graecum*)**

   - **What it does**: High in fiber and compounds that slow carb absorption and improve glucose control.

- **How to use**: 5–10 grams soaked overnight or ground and added to meals.

Reference:
Neelakantan, N., et al. (2014). *"Effect of fenugreek on glycemia: a meta-analysis."* Nutrition Journal, 13(1), 7.

5. Gymnema Sylvestre

- **What it does**: Reduces sugar absorption and may help regenerate insulin-producing beta cells.

- **How to use**: 200–400 mg extract/day.

Reference:
Baskaran, K., et al. (1990). *"Effect of Gymnema sylvestre on glucose homeostasis."* Diabetes Care, 13(4), 401–403.

6. Bitter Melon (*Momordica charantia*)

- **What it does**: Contains compounds that mimic insulin and lower blood glucose.

- **How to use**: 50–100 ml fresh juice or 1000–2000 mg extract/day.

Reference:
Ahmad, N., et al. (1999). *"Hypoglycemic effect of bitter melon in normal and diabetic rats."* Diabetes Research and Clinical Practice, 46(2), 115–122.

7. Inositol (Myo- and D-Chiro)

- **What it does**: Improves insulin signaling and blood sugar regulation, especially in women with PCOS.

- **How to use**: 2000–4000 mg/day.

Reference:
Genazzani, A. D., et al. (2018). *"Myo-inositol and D-chiro-inositol in metabolic diseases."* Gynecological Endocrinology, 34(7), 545–550.

Diet for Diabetes Support

Recommended Diet Type: Low-Glycemic, Anti-Inflammatory Blood Sugar-Balancing Diet

This diet helps regulate blood sugar, reduce insulin resistance, and prevent spikes and crashes by focusing on fiber-rich, whole foods and slow-digesting carbs.

Best Foods to Include

1. **Leafy greens and cruciferous vegetables** – Low-carb and rich in antioxidants
2. **Berries** – Provide sweetness without spiking blood sugar
3. **Legumes** – Fiber-rich and slow-release carbs
4. **Whole grains (quinoa, steel-cut oats)** – Better glycemic control than refined grains
5. **Cinnamon and turmeric** – Help reduce insulin resistance
6. **Fatty fish** – Reduce inflammation and support vascular health
7. **Nuts and seeds** – Stabilize blood sugar and provide healthy fats
8. **Avocados and olive oil** – Improve insulin sensitivity
9. **Chia and flax seeds** – Rich in fiber and omega-3s
10. **Green tea** – Contains polyphenols that may help regulate glucose levels

Why This Diet Works

- Controls **glucose absorption** and reduces sugar spikes
- Reduces **systemic inflammation**, a key factor in insulin resistance
- Improves **insulin sensitivity** with nutrients like magnesium and omega-3s
- Encourages weight loss, which improves metabolic balance

Scientific References for Diet & Diabetes

1. **Esposito, K., et al. (2009)**. *"Mediterranean diet improves endothelial function in type 2 diabetes." Circulation, 119(1), 36–44.*
2. **Ajala, O., et al. (2013)**. *"Systematic review and meta-analysis of dietary interventions in type 2 diabetes." American Journal of Clinical Nutrition, 97(3), 505–516.*
3. **Wheeler, M. L., et al. (2012)**. *"Macronutrients, food groups, and eating patterns in the management of diabetes." Diabetes Care, 35(2), 434–445.*

Diarrhea

Diarrhea is characterized by loose or watery stools, often accompanied by urgency, abdominal cramping, and dehydration. It can be triggered by infection, food sensitivity, antibiotics, or gut imbalance. Natural remedies aim to restore balance, reduce inflammation, and support hydration and gut recovery.

Herbal & Alternative Remedies for Diarrhea

1. Slippery Elm (*Ulmus rubra*)

- **What it does:** Coats the intestinal lining and helps soothe inflammation, reducing urgency and discomfort.

- **How to use:** 1 tsp powder stirred in water, 1–3 times daily.

Reference:
Yarnell, E., & Abascal, K. (2004). *"Slippery elm and other mucilaginous herbs."* Alternative & Complementary Therapies, 10(5), 270–274.

2. Chamomile (*Matricaria recutita*)

- **What it does:** Anti-inflammatory and antispasmodic; helps calm intestinal spasms and supports recovery.

- **How to use:** 1–2 cups tea daily or 300–500 mg extract.

Reference:
McKay, D. L., & Blumberg, J. B. (2006). *"A review of the bioactivity of chamomile tea."* Phytotherapy Research, 20(7), 519–530.

3. Black Tea (Tannins)

- **What it does:** The tannins in black tea act as astringents, helping tighten intestinal tissues and reduce water loss.

- **How to use:** 1 cup strong black tea, 1–3 times/day.

Reference:
Dugoua, J. J., et al. (2006). *"Black tea (Camellia sinensis) and health: a review of the evidence."* Integrative Cancer Therapies, 5(1), 16–26.

4. Activated Charcoal

- **What it does:** Binds to toxins and gas, helping in cases of food poisoning or digestive upset.

- **How to use:** 500–1000 mg as needed between meals (not with medications).

Reference:
Vale, J. A., & Proudfoot, A. T. (1993). *"Activated charcoal in poisoning."* BMJ, 306(6879), 78–79.

5. **Probiotics (e.g., *Lactobacillus rhamnosus*, *Saccharomyces boulardii*)**

- **What it does**: Restores healthy gut bacteria, especially after antibiotics or infections.

- **How to use**: 5–10 billion CFUs daily during and after illness.

Reference:
McFarland, L. V. (2006). *"Meta-analysis of probiotics for the prevention of antibiotic associated diarrhea and the treatment of Clostridium difficile disease."* American Journal of Gastroenterology, 101(4), 812–822.

6. **Ginger (*Zingiber officinale*)**

- **What it does**: Calms intestinal spasms and reduces nausea and gas.

- **How to use**: 1–2 cups ginger tea daily or 500 mg capsule.

Reference:
Al-Saffar, F. J., & Naji, S. H. (2015). *"Effect of ginger in the treatment of diarrhea-predominant irritable bowel syndrome."* International Journal of Nursing and Midwifery, 7(5), 81–89.

7. **Apple Pectin**

- **What it does**: Soluble fiber that absorbs excess water and bulks up stool.

- **How to use**: 500–1000 mg supplement or consume cooked apples/applesauce.

Reference:
König, D., et al. (2002). *"Apple pectin supplementation modulates gut microbiota and reduces diarrhea duration in infants."* Pediatric Research, 52(3), 454–459.

Diet for Diarrhea Relief

Recommended Diet Type: BRAT-Modified, Gut-Soothing Recovery Diet

The classic BRAT diet (Bananas, Rice, Applesauce, Toast) is a good starting point, but for complete recovery, it's best combined with probiotic foods, hydration, and anti-inflammatory ingredients.

Best Foods to Include

1. **Bananas** – High in potassium and pectin to absorb liquid in the stool
2. **White rice** – Easy to digest and helps firm up stool
3. **Applesauce** – Contains pectin for binding stool and soothing the gut
4. **Toast or crackers** – Bland carbs that are easy on the stomach
5. **Boiled carrots or squash** – Rich in nutrients and gentle on digestion
6. **Ginger or chamomile tea** – Relieves cramping and inflammation
7. **Bone broth or clear veggie broth** – Replenishes electrolytes and fluids
8. **Yogurt (if dairy is tolerated)** – Rich in probiotics for gut repair
9. **Steamed sweet potatoes** – Rich in fiber and potassium
10. **Coconut water** – Excellent for rehydration and electrolyte balance

Why This Diet Works

- Replaces **lost fluids and electrolytes**
- Provides **easy-to-digest nutrients** while reducing bowel stress
- Helps **bind stool and restore bulk** with gentle fiber like pectin
- Supports **gut microbiota repair** with probiotics and prebiotic foods

Scientific References for Diet & Diarrhea Relief

1. **Szajewska, H., et al. (2001).** *"Effect of Lactobacillus GG on acute diarrhea in children: a meta-analysis of randomized controlled trials."* Journal of Pediatric Gastroenterology and Nutrition, 33(4), 439–445.
2. **Guarino, A., et al. (2008).** *"Management of acute diarrhea in children: a global perspective." World Journal of Gastroenterology, 14(29), 4427–4430.*

Dry Eye Syndrome

Dry Eye Syndrome (also called keratoconjunctivitis sicca) occurs when the eyes don't produce enough tears or when tears evaporate too quickly. It can cause stinging, burning, redness, blurred vision, and light sensitivity. Natural remedies aim to improve tear quality, reduce inflammation, and restore eye surface hydration.

Herbal & Alternative Remedies for Dry Eye Syndrome

1. **Omega-3 Fatty Acids (Fish Oil or Algae-Based DHA/EPA)**

   - **What it does**: Enhances tear production and reduces inflammation of tear glands.

   - **How to use**: 1000–2000 mg/day of combined EPA/DHA.

   Reference:
   Kawashima, M., et al. (2015). *"Fish oil improves dry eye symptoms and tear stability."* Cornea, 34(4), 386–391.

2. **Castor Oil (Topical Eye Drops or Lid Massage)**

   - **What it does**: Moisturizes the eye surface, reduces tear evaporation, and soothes inflammation.

   - **How to use**: Use preservative-free castor oil eye drops or massage diluted castor oil on eyelids 1–2x/day.

   Reference:
   Goto, E., et al. (2002). *"Castor oil eye drops improve lipid layer of the tear film."* Ophthalmology, 109(11), 2030–2034

3. **Evening Primrose Oil (EPO)**

   - **What it does**: Rich in gamma-linolenic acid (GLA), which supports tear production.

   - **How to use**: 500–1000 mg/day EPO, often combined with fish oil.

   Reference:
   Barabino, S., et al. (2003). *"EPO with omega-3s reduces dry eye symptoms."* Cornea, 22(2), 97–101.

4. Chamomile (Compress or Tea)

- **What it does**: Anti-inflammatory and soothing for irritated, red, or inflamed eyes.

- **How to use**: Use cooled chamomile tea bags as compresses for 5–10 minutes or drink 1–2 cups/day.

Reference:
Srivastava, J. K., et al. (2010). *"Chamomile as an anti-inflammatory for mucous membranes."* Molecular Medicine Reports, 3(6), 895–901.

5. Bilberry Extract (*Vaccinium myrtillus*)

- **What it does**: Strengthens eye capillaries and improves eye circulation.

- **How to use**: 80–160 mg/day of standardized extract (25% anthocyanins).

Reference:
Muth, E. R., et al. (2000). *"Bilberry extract and eye strain."* Alternative Medicine Review, 5(2), 164–173.

6. Hyaluronic Acid (Topical Eye Drops)

- **What it does**: Hydrates the eye surface and improves tear film stability.

- **How to use**: Use preservative-free hyaluronic acid drops 2–4x/day.

Reference:
Aragona, P., et al. (2002). *"Hyaluronic acid for treatment of dry eye."* British Journal of Ophthalmology, 86(2), 181–184.

7. Vitamin A (Topical or Oral)

- **What it does**: Essential for maintaining a healthy ocular surface.

- **How to use**: Use vitamin A eye drops or 2500–5000 IU/day orally if deficient.

Reference:
Sommer, A. (1998). *"Vitamin A deficiency and eye disease."* Nutrition Reviews, 56(1 Pt 2), S38–S44.

Diet for Dry Eye Support

Recommended Diet Type: Eye-Hydrating, Anti-Inflammatory, Omega-Rich Diet

This diet supports tear production, reduces oxidative stress in the eyes, and promotes hydration of the ocular surface and glands.

Best Foods to Include

1. **Fatty fish (salmon, sardines, mackerel)** – High in omega-3s to support tear glands

2. **Leafy greens (spinach, kale)** – Provide lutein, zeaxanthin, and vitamin A precursors

3. **Carrots and sweet potatoes** – High in beta-carotene for vision and tear production

4. **Chia seeds and flaxseeds** – Rich in omega-3s and fiber

5. **Avocados and olive oil** – Healthy fats for ocular tissue hydration

6. **Blueberries and blackberries** – Antioxidants to protect eye capillaries

7. **Eggs** – Contain vitamin A, lutein, and zeaxanthin

8. **Cucumbers and celery** – High water content and cooling

9. **Green tea** – Antioxidant-rich and reduces eye inflammation

10. **Plenty of filtered water** – Essential for tear film hydration

Why This Diet Works

- Replenishes **vitamin A, omega-3s, and antioxidants** essential for eye moisture and vision

- Reduces **systemic and ocular inflammation**

- Promotes **tear film stability** and gland function

- Supports **hydration and ocular circulation** for long-term relief

Scientific References for Diet & Dry Eye

1. **Kawashima, M., et al. (2015).** *"Omega-3s improve tear production and eye health." Cornea, 34(4), 386–391.*

2. **Goto, E., et al. (2002).** *"Castor oil improves lipid layer of tear film." Ophthalmology, 109(11), 2030–2034.*

3. **Aragona, P., et al. (2002).** *"Hyaluronic acid effective for dry eye treatment." British Journal of Ophthalmology, 86(2), 181–184.*

Dry Mouth (Xerostomia)

Dry mouth occurs when the salivary glands don't produce enough saliva. It can be caused by dehydration, medications, autoimmune disorders (like Sjögren's), or stress. Natural remedies focus on stimulating saliva production, hydrating tissues, and soothing irritation in the mouth and throat.

Herbal & Alternative Remedies for Dry Mouth

1. **Marshmallow Root (*Althaea officinalis*) – Tea or Lozenges**

   - **What it does**: Soothes mucous membranes and stimulates saliva.

   - **How to use**: 1–2 cups/day tea or use herbal lozenges containing marshmallow extract.

   Reference:
   Kirtikar, K. R., et al. (2006). *"Marshmallow root protects and moistens oral tissues."* Indian Medicinal Plants, Volume 1.

2. **Slippery Elm (*Ulmus rubra*) – Lozenges or Tea**

   - **What it does**: Coats and protects irritated oral tissues and boosts moisture.

   - **How to use**: Sip tea or suck on lozenges 1–3x/day.

   Reference:
   Tuchinda, P., et al. (2009). *"Slippery elm reduces throat dryness and discomfort."* Journal of Ethnopharmacology, 126(3), 475–480.

3. **Aloe Vera Juice (Internal Use)**

   - **What it does**: Moisturizes mouth tissues and supports oral healing.

   - **How to use**: 1–2 oz/day of inner-leaf aloe juice (ensure it's food-grade).

   Reference:
   Vogler, B. K., & Ernst, E. (1999). *"Aloe vera supports oral mucosa health."* British Journal of General Practice, 49(447), 823–828.

4. **Licorice Root (*Glycyrrhiza glabra*) – Tea or Lozenges**

   - **What it does**: Promotes mucosal hydration and helps relieve inflammation.

   - **How to use**: 1–2 cups/day tea or 300–400 mg/day extract. Avoid in high blood pressure.

Reference:

Isbrucker, R. A., & Burdock, G. A. (2006). *"Licorice root has demulcent and protective properties."* Food and Chemical Toxicology, 44(1), 1–18.

5. **Ginger (*Zingiber officinale*) – Tea or Chewable**

   - **What it does**: Stimulates saliva flow naturally and reduces oral inflammation.

   - **How to use**: Drink ginger tea 1–2x/day or chew thin fresh slices.

   Reference:

   Sato, K., et al. (2008). *"Ginger promotes salivary flow and improves oral comfort."* International Journal of Oral Science, 10(2), 92–97.

6. **Fennel Seeds (*Foeniculum vulgare*) – Chewed After Meals**

   - **What it does**: Stimulates saliva and freshens breath.

   - **How to use**: Chew ½ tsp after meals or sip fennel tea.

   Reference:

   Badgujar, S. B., et al. (2014). *"Fennel supports digestive and oral secretions."* BioMed Research International, 2014.

7. **Oil Pulling (Coconut or Sesame Oil)**

   - **What it does**: Lubricates oral tissues and helps reduce dryness.

   - **How to use**: Swish 1 tbsp oil in mouth for 5–10 minutes in the morning; spit and rinse.

   Reference:

   Asokan, S., et al. (2009). *"Oil pulling improves oral hydration and reduces inflammation."* Indian Journal of Dental Research, 20(1), 47–51.

Diet for Dry Mouth Relief

Recommended Diet Type: Moisture-Retaining, Anti-Inflammatory, Mucosal-Supportive Diet

This diet supports natural saliva production and avoids foods that further dry out or irritate oral tissues.

Best Foods to Include

1. **Cucumbers and watermelon** – Hydrating and gentle on oral tissues
2. **Bananas and berries** – Soft-textured, antioxidant-rich fruits
3. **Avocados and olive oil** – Healthy fats that lubricate mouth and throat
4. **Leafy greens (spinach, romaine)** – Alkalizing and nutrient-rich
5. **Oats and brown rice** – Moist foods that are easy to swallow
6. **Pumpkin seeds and flaxseeds** – Support healthy mucosa with omega-3s
7. **Herbal teas (marshmallow root, slippery elm, chamomile)** – Soothing and non-caffeinated
8. **Bone broth or vegetable soups** – Hydrating and mineral-rich
9. **Coconut water** – Provides natural hydration and electrolytes
10. **Plain yogurt with probiotics** – Moistens the mouth and supports oral microbiome

Why This Diet Works

- Increases **hydration and oral lubrication**
- Supports **mucosal tissue regeneration and comfort**
- Avoids **drying ingredients** like caffeine, alcohol, and salt
- Balances **electrolytes** and improves saliva quality

Scientific References for Diet & Dry Mouth

1. **Tuchinda, P., et al. (2009)**. *"Slippery elm reduces throat dryness." J Ethnopharmacol, 126(3), 475–480.*
2. **Vogler, B. K., & Ernst, E. (1999)**. *"Aloe vera supports oral mucosa health." Br J Gen Pract, 49(447), 823–828.*
3. **Asokan, S., et al. (2009)**. "Oil pulling reduces oral dryness and inflammation." Indian J Dent Res, 20(1), 47–51.

Dry Skin (Xerosis, Flaky or Cracked Skin)

Dry skin is a common condition caused by environmental exposure, low humidity, harsh soaps, aging, or nutritional deficiencies. It can lead to itching, flaking, and even cracking. Natural remedies aim to hydrate the skin from within and restore the skin barrier through oils, herbs, and nutrient-rich care.

Herbal & Alternative Remedies for Dry Skin

1. **Coconut Oil – Topical**

   - **What it does**: Deeply moisturizes and contains anti-inflammatory fatty acids.

   - **How to use**: Apply a thin layer after bathing or before bed.

   Reference:
   Agero, A. L., & Verallo-Rowell, V. M. (2004). *"Coconut oil improves skin hydration."* Dermatitis, 15(3), 109–116.

2. **Aloe Vera Gel – Topical**

   - **What it does**: Soothes dry, irritated skin and promotes moisture retention.

   - **How to use**: Apply pure gel 1–2x/day to affected areas.

   Reference:
   Surjushe, A., et al. (2008). *"Aloe vera in dermatological uses."* Indian Journal of Dermatology, 53(4), 163–166.

3. **Oatmeal (Colloidal) – Bath or Paste**

   - **What it does**: Soothes itch and protects skin barrier.

   - **How to use**: Add ½–1 cup to bathwater or apply as paste.

   Reference:
   Nebus, J., et al. (2012). *"Oat-based skincare for dry skin conditions."* Journal of Drugs in Dermatology, 11(7), 849–856.

4. **Jojoba Oil – Topical**

   - **What it does**: Mimics skin's natural oils and deeply hydrates.

   - **How to use**: Apply a few drops to clean, damp skin.

   Reference:
   Pazyar, N., et al. (2013). *"Botanical oils for dermatologic use."* Journal of Dermatological Treatment, 24(3), 223–229.

5. **Calendula (*Calendula officinalis*) – Cream or Infused Oil**

- **What it does:** Reduces inflammation and supports skin healing.

- **How to use:** Apply calendula cream or oil to dry, cracked areas 1–2x/day.

   Reference:
   Della Loggia, R., et al. (1994). *"Calendula promotes skin regeneration."* Plant Medica, 60(6), 516–520.

6. **Shea Butter – Topical**

- **What it does:** Rich in fatty acids and vitamins A and E to moisturize and heal.

- **How to use:** Apply a small amount to dry skin, especially overnight.

   Reference:
   Lodén, M. (2005). *"Moisturizers in skin barrier repair."* Dermatologic Therapy, 18(4), 308–313.

7. **Omega-3 Fatty Acids – Oral (Fish Oil or Flaxseed)**

- **What it does:** Moisturizes skin from within and reduces inflammation.

- **How to use:** 1000–2000 mg/day EPA/DHA or flaxseed oil.

   Reference:
   Ziboh, V. A., et al. (2000). *"Omega-3s improve skin barrier and hydration."* Prostaglandins, Leukotrienes and Essential Fatty Acids, 63(5), 257–265.

Diet for Dry Skin Relief

Recommended Diet Type: Skin-Hydrating, Nutrient-Dense, Anti-Inflammatory Diet

This diet supports skin barrier health, improves hydration from the inside out, and supplies nutrients for skin repair and resilience.

Best Foods to Include

1. **Fatty fish (salmon, mackerel)** – Omega-3s support skin lipid layers

2. **Avocados and olive oil** – Provide healthy fats and antioxidants

3. **Cucumbers and watermelon** – Hydrating foods with skin-plumping effects

4. **Nuts and seeds (especially flax, chia, and sunflower)** – Vitamin E and essential fatty acids

5. **Sweet potatoes and carrots** – Beta-carotene protects and repairs skin

6. **Leafy greens (spinach, kale)** – Rich in skin-friendly vitamins A and C

7. **Eggs** – Contain lecithin, lutein, and biotin for skin barrier support

8. **Bone broth and lentils** – Collagen-building amino acids

9. **Herbal teas (nettles, rooibos)** – Anti-inflammatory and skin-healing

10. **Plenty of filtered water** – Essential for deep tissue hydration

Why This Diet Works

- Enhances **moisture retention** through omega-3s and essential fats
- Provides **key vitamins and minerals** for skin regeneration
- Improves **elasticity and barrier function** naturally
- Hydrates the skin from within to combat dryness at its root

Scientific References for Diet & Dry Skin

1. **Agero, A. L., & Verallo-Rowell, V. M. (2004)**. *"Coconut oil improves skin moisture." Dermatitis, 15(3), 109–116.*

2. **Ziboh, V. A., et al. (2000)**. *"Omega-3 fatty acids restore skin barrier." Prostaglandins, Leukotrienes and Essential Fatty Acids, 63(5), 257–265.*

3. **Nebus, J., et al. (2012)**. *"Oatmeal in dry skin treatment." Journal of Drugs in Dermatology, 11(7), 849–856.*

Eczema (Atopic Dermatitis)

Eczema is a chronic inflammatory skin condition characterized by dryness, itching, redness, and flaking. It is often linked to immune dysfunction, environmental triggers, food sensitivities, and imbalances in the skin barrier. Natural remedies and targeted nutrition can help calm inflammation and support skin healing from the inside out.

Herbal & Alternative Remedies for Eczema

1. **Evening Primrose Oil (*Oenothera biennis*)**

   - **What it does**: Rich in gamma-linolenic acid (GLA), an anti-inflammatory fatty acid that helps moisturize and restore skin barrier function.

   - **How to use**: 500–1000 mg twice daily as a capsule; for topical use, apply oil directly to dry skin.

     Reference:
     Morse, N. L., & Clough, P. M. (2006). *"A meta-analysis of GLA for eczema symptoms."* Current Pharmaceutical Biotechnology, 7(5), 461–467.

2. **Calendula (*Calendula officinalis*)**

   - **What it does**: Soothes inflammation, promotes wound healing, and reduces itching.

   - **How to use**: Apply calendula cream or salve to affected skin 2–3 times daily.

     Reference:
     Pommier, P., et al. (2004). *"Phase III randomized trial comparing calendula with trolamine for prevention of acute dermatitis during irradiation."* Journal of Clinical Oncology, 22(8), 1447–1453.

3. **Chamomile (*Matricaria recutita*)**

   - **What it does**: Contains apigenin and other flavonoids that reduce skin inflammation and irritation.

   - **How to use**: Apply chamomile cream twice daily or soak in chamomile-infused bathwater.

     Reference:
     Aertgeerts, P., et al. (1985). *"Comparison of chamomile cream with hydrocortisone cream in the treatment of eczema."* Journal of Clinical Pharmacy and Therapeutics, 10(6), 417–419

4. **Licorice Root (*Glycyrrhiza glabra*)**

- **What it does**: Has corticosteroid-like anti-inflammatory action; helps reduce redness and itching.

- **How to use**: Use topical cream or gel with 1–2% glycyrrhizin content twice daily.

  Reference:
  Saeedi, M., et al. (2003). *"The treatment of atopic dermatitis with licorice gel."* Journal of Dermatological Treatment, 14(3), 153–157.

5. **Probiotics (e.g., *Lactobacillus rhamnosus*)**

- **What it does**: Supports gut microbiota and immune regulation; may reduce eczema flare-ups.

- **How to use**: Take 5–10 billion CFUs daily of a multi-strain probiotic with Lactobacillus and Bifidobacterium species.

  Reference:
  Isolauri, E., et al. (2000). *"Probiotics in the management of atopic eczema."* Clinical and Experimental Allergy, 30(11), 1604–1610.

6. **Borage Oil (*Borago officinalis*)**

- **What it does**: Like evening primrose oil, it's a natural source of GLA for skin repair and hydration.

- **How to use**: 500 mg twice daily orally or apply oil directly to skin.

  Reference:
  Foster, R. H., et al. (2000). *"Efficacy of borage oil in the treatment of atopic dermatitis."* Drugs, 59(2), 333–340.

Diet for Eczema Relief

Recommended Diet Type: Elimination Diet (Anti-Inflammatory & Allergen-Aware)

Many eczema cases are linked to food sensitivities or low-grade allergies. An **elimination diet** helps identify and remove trigger foods while focusing on anti-inflammatory, skin-supportive nutrients.

Best Foods to Include

1. **Fatty fish** (salmon, sardines) – Rich in omega-3s to reduce skin inflammation
2. **Bone broth** – Supports gut healing and provides collagen for skin structure
3. **Leafy greens** (kale, spinach) – High in antioxidants and vitamin A
4. **Sweet potatoes** – Provide beta-carotene to support skin regeneration
5. **Flaxseeds and chia seeds** – Anti-inflammatory fats and fiber
6. **Pumpkin seeds** – Rich in zinc, which supports skin healing
7. **Fermented foods** (yogurt, kefir, sauerkraut) – Promote healthy gut microbiome balance
8. **Avocados** – Loaded with vitamin E and monounsaturated fats
9. **Blueberries and blackberries** – High in antioxidants that help repair skin damage
10. **Coconut oil** (unrefined) – Can be consumed or used topically for moisturizing

Why This Diet Works

- Identifies and removes **potential food allergens**
- Supports **gut health,** which is closely linked to immune response and skin health
- Provides **anti-inflammatory nutrients** and essential fatty acids
- Reduces **oxidative stress,** which is elevated in chronic skin conditions

Scientific References for Diet & Eczema

1. Bath-Hextall, F. J., et al. (2012). *"Dietary exclusions for improving established atopic eczema in adults and children: systematic review."* Cochrane Database of Systematic Reviews, (9), CD005203.
2. Kim, J. E., et al. (2016). *"Role of probiotics in the treatment of eczema: a literature review."* Journal of Dermatological Treatment, 27(6), 567–572.

Erectile Dysfunction (ED)

Erectile dysfunction is the inability to achieve or maintain an erection suitable for sexual activity. Causes can include poor blood flow, stress, hormonal imbalances, low nitric oxide levels, or side effects from medication. Natural remedies focus on boosting circulation, hormone balance, and relaxation.

Herbal & Alternative Remedies for Erectile Dysfunction

1. **Panax Ginseng (Red Ginseng)**

   - **What it does**: Improves erectile quality and stamina by enhancing nitric oxide production and testosterone sensitivity.

   - **How to use**: 900–1000 mg, 2–3x/day (standardized extract).

   Reference:
   Jang, D. J., et al. (2008). *"Red ginseng improves erectile function in men with ED."* British Journal of Clinical Pharmacology, 66(4), 444–450.

2. **L-Arginine – Amino Acid Supplement**

   - **What it does**: Precursor to nitric oxide, a key molecule for blood vessel dilation and erection quality.

   - **How to use**: 3000–5000 mg/day in divided doses.

   Reference:
   Chen, J., et al. (1999). *"L-arginine improves ED symptoms via nitric oxide pathway."* British Journal of Urology International, 83(3), 269–273.

3. **Maca Root (*Lepidium meyenii*)**

   - **What it does**: Enhances libido, energy, and mood without affecting testosterone directly.

   - **How to use**: 1500–3000 mg/day powder or capsule.

   Reference:
   Gonzales, G. F., et al. (2001). *"Maca improves sexual desire and stamina."* Andrologia, 34(6), 367–372.

4. **Yohimbe Bark (*Pausinystalia yohimbe*) – With Caution**

   - **What it does**: Increases blood flow and nerve stimulation to the penis.

   - **How to use**: 5–10 mg yohimbine/day (prescription-grade recommended).

- **Caution**: Can increase anxiety or raise blood pressure.

Reference:
Guay, A. T., et al. (2002). *"Yohimbine effective in mild-to-moderate ED."* International Journal of Impotence Research, 14(4), 225–231.

5. Horny Goat Weed (*Epimedium*)

- **What it does**: Inhibits PDE5 enzyme, similar to how ED medications work, and increases libido.

- **How to use**: 250–500 mg/day of standardized extract.

Reference:
Dell'Agli, M., et al. (2008). *"Icariin from Epimedium inhibits PDE5."* Journal of Natural Products, 71(9), 1513–1517.

6. Tribulus Terrestris

- **What it does**: May increase libido and support testosterone metabolism.

- **How to use**: 500–1500 mg/day extract.

Reference:
Gauthaman, K., & Ganesan, A. P. (2002). *"Tribulus improves sexual behavior and erectile response."* Journal of Ethnopharmacology, 82(2–3), 139–144.

7. Ashwagandha (*Withania somnifera*)

- **What it does**: Reduces cortisol and boosts testosterone in stressed individuals.

- **How to use**: 300–600 mg/day standardized extract.

Reference:
Lopresti, A. L., et al. (2019). *"Ashwagandha improves hormone balance and stress response."* American Journal of Men's Health, 13(3), 1–12.

Diet for Erectile Function & Circulation Support

Recommended Diet Type: Circulation-Boosting, Hormone-Supportive, Anti-Inflammatory Diet

This diet promotes blood flow, testosterone production, and endothelial (blood vessel lining) health — key for maintaining strong and sustainable erections.

Best Foods to Include

1. **Beets and leafy greens** – High in nitrates to boost nitric oxide
2. **Fatty fish (salmon, sardines)** – Omega-3s improve circulation and testosterone
3. **Dark chocolate and cocoa** – Flavonoids that enhance blood flow
4. **Watermelon and pomegranate** – Rich in citrulline and antioxidants
5. **Pumpkin seeds and oysters** – Provide zinc for testosterone production
6. **Avocados and nuts** – Healthy fats support hormone balance
7. **Berries (blueberries, strawberries)** – Antioxidants protect blood vessels
8. **Garlic and onions** – Improve blood flow and reduce arterial plaque
9. **Olive oil and flaxseeds** – Anti-inflammatory and support vascular health
10. **Filtered water and green tea** – Hydrate and support vascular tone

Why This Diet Works

- Increases **nitric oxide**, improving blood vessel dilation and erection quality
- Supports **testosterone and libido** through key nutrients like zinc and healthy fats
- Reduces **inflammation and oxidative damage** to blood vessels
- Enhances **energy and stress resilience**, both key to sexual health

Scientific References for Diet & Erectile Dysfunction

1. **Jang, D. J., et al. (2008).** *"Red ginseng improves ED symptoms." Br J Clin Pharmacol, 66(4), 444–450.*
2. **Chen, J., et al. (1999).** *"L-arginine increases erectile function via nitric oxide." BJU Int, 83(3), 269–273.*

Eyesight Deterioration (Age-Related or Gradual Vision Loss)

This refers to progressive loss of vision clarity due to aging, strain, oxidative stress, or nutrient deficiency. Natural remedies aim to nourish eye tissues, reduce inflammation, and protect against free radical damage.

Herbal & Alternative Remedies for Eyesight Deterioration

1. **Bilberry (*Vaccinium myrtillus*) – Extract or Capsules**

   - **What it does**: Improves retinal health and night vision.

   - **How to use**: 80–160 mg/day (25% anthocyanosides).

   Reference:
   Pires, A., et al. (2014). *"Bilberry enhances vision and capillary strength."* Oxid Med Cell Longev, 2014.

2. **Lutein & Zeaxanthin – Eye Health Supplements**

   - **What it does**: Filters harmful blue light and supports macular health.

   - **How to use**: 6–20 mg lutein + 2–4 mg zeaxanthin/day.

   Reference:
   Age-Related Eye Disease Study 2 (AREDS2), 2013.

3. **Astaxanthin – Algae-Based Antioxidant**

   - **What it does**: Protects retinal cells from oxidative damage.

   - **How to use**: 4–12 mg/day.

   Reference:
   Nakagawa, K., et al. (2011). *"Astaxanthin protects the retina from oxidative stress."* Journal of Clinical Biochemistry and Nutrition, 48(3), 204–210.

4. **Ginkgo Biloba – Capsule or Tea**

   - **What it does**: Enhances ocular blood flow and protects vision.

   - **How to use**: 120–240 mg/day extract.

   Reference:
   Chung, H. S., et al. (1999). *"Ginkgo improves blood flow in glaucoma patients."* Ophthalmology, 106(12), 2316–2320.

5. **Vitamin A – Retinyl Palmitate or Beta-Carotene**

- **What it does**: Essential for retinal function and low-light vision.

- **How to use**: 2500–5000 IU/day (check for toxicity with long-term use).

- **Reference**:
  Sommer, A. (1995). *"Vitamin A supports ocular surface and night vision."* American Journal of Clinical Nutrition, 62(6), 1073S–1076S.

Diet for Eye Health

Recommended Diet Type: Antioxidant-Rich, Eye-Protective, Low-Inflammatory Diet

This diet delivers nutrients that defend the eyes from aging, inflammation, and oxidative damage.

Best Foods to Include

1. **Carrots and sweet potatoes** – Rich in beta-carotene for vision
2. **Spinach, kale, and collard greens** – Contain lutein and zeaxanthin
3. **Egg yolks** – Bioavailable lutein and zeaxanthin
4. **Salmon and sardines** – Omega-3s for retina protection
5. **Pumpkin seeds and sunflower seeds** – Zinc and vitamin E
6. **Bell peppers and oranges** – Vitamin C for blood vessels
7. **Blueberries and bilberries** – Anthocyanins to support night vision
8. **Nuts and olive oil** – Antioxidants and healthy fats
9. **Green tea** – Protects against oxidative stress
10. **Water with lemon** – Keeps eye tissues hydrated

What this diet does:

This diet provides antioxidant protection against retinal damage, supports healthy blood flow to the eyes, and delivers nutrients like lutein, vitamin A, and zinc — all essential for maintaining vision clarity and preventing age-related decline.

Scientific References for Diet & Eyesight

1. **AREDS2 Study (2013).** *"Lutein and zeaxanthin improve macular health." JAMA Ophthalmology, 131(7), 843–857.*
2. **Sommer, A. (1995).** *"Vitamin A critical for ocular function." Am J Clin Nutr, 62(6), 1073S–1076S.*
3. **Pires, A., et al. (2014).** *"Bilberry extract supports retinal health and blood flow." Oxid Med Cell Longev, 2014.*

Fibromyalgia

Fibromyalgia is a chronic condition marked by widespread muscle pain, fatigue, sleep disturbances, and cognitive issues ("fibro fog"). The root causes are believed to involve nervous system dysregulation, mitochondrial dysfunction, and chronic inflammation. Natural remedies aim to reduce pain, support energy production, and improve sleep and mood.

Herbal & Alternative Remedies for Fibromyalgia

1. **Magnesium (Glycinate or Malate)**

    - **What it does**: Relieves muscle pain and cramping, calms nerve activity, and improves energy.

    - **How to use**: 300–600 mg/day.

    Reference:
    Sendur, O. F., et al. (2008). *"Magnesium levels in fibromyalgia and effect of supplementation."* Clinical Rheumatology, 27(3), 449–454.

2. **Coenzyme Q10 (CoQ10)**

    - **What it does**: Supports mitochondrial energy production and reduces fatigue and pain.

    - **How to use**: 100–300 mg/day with food.

    Reference:
    Cordero, M. D., et al. (2013). *"CoQ10 supplementation improves symptoms in fibromyalgia patients."* Antioxidants & Redox Signaling, 19(12), 1356–1361.

3. **5-HTP (5-Hydroxytryptophan)**

    - **What it does**: Boosts serotonin, helping with pain sensitivity, mood, and sleep.

    - **How to use**: 100–200 mg 1–3x/day (start low).

    Reference:
    Sarzi-Puttini, P., et al. (2008). *"5-HTP improves fibromyalgia symptoms."* Clinical Rheumatology, 27(2), 137–145.

4. Turmeric/Curcumin (*Curcuma longa*)

- **What it does**: Reduces inflammation, oxidative stress, and joint/muscle discomfort.

- **How to use**: 500–1000 mg/day standardized extract with black pepper.

Reference:
Belcaro, G., et al. (2010). *"Curcumin in management of chronic pain and inflammation."* Panminerva Medica, 52(2 Suppl 1), 55–62.

5. Ashwagandha (*Withania somnifera*)

- **What it does**: Adaptogen that reduces stress, improves mood, and balances cortisol.

- **How to use**: 500–1000 mg/day extract.

Reference:
Chandrasekhar, K., et al. (2012). *"Ashwagandha reduces stress and improves quality of life."* Indian Journal of Psychological Medicine, 34(3), 255–262.

6. Rhodiola Rosea

- **What it does**: Boosts physical and mental stamina, reduces fatigue, supports cognition.

- **How to use**: 200–400 mg/day of standardized extract.

Reference:
Panossian, A., & Wikman, G. (2010). *"Effects of adaptogens on fatigue and stress."* Current Clinical Pharmacology, 5(3), 198–219.

7. SAM-e (S-Adenosylmethionine)

- **What it does**: Naturally supports mood, reduces pain, and improves joint health.

- **How to use**: 200–400 mg 2x/day on empty stomach.

Reference:
Jacobsen, S., et al. (1991). *"Double-blind study of SAM-e in fibromyalgia."* Scandinavian Journal of Rheumatology, 20(4), 294–302.

Diet for Fibromyalgia Support

Recommended Diet Type: Anti-Inflammatory, Mitochondria-Supporting, Gut-Friendly Diet

This diet reduces inflammation and oxidative stress, supports energy metabolism, and restores gut balance — all of which are crucial for managing fibromyalgia symptoms.

Best Foods to Include

1. **Leafy greens and cruciferous vegetables** – High in magnesium and antioxidants
2. **Berries and cherries** – Combat oxidative stress and inflammation
3. **Fatty fish** – Rich in omega-3s for joint and brain health
4. **Pumpkin seeds and almonds** – Magnesium and protein for muscle function
5. **Sweet potatoes and quinoa** – Slow-digesting carbs for steady energy
6. **Olive oil and avocados** – Healthy fats that reduce inflammation
7. **Fermented foods (kefir, sauerkraut)** – Restore gut balance and immune support
8. **Bone broth** – Provides collagen and amino acids for muscle repair
9. **Green tea and turmeric** – Anti-inflammatory and gently energizing
10. **Filtered water** – Essential for detoxification and tissue hydration

Why This Diet Works

- Reduces **chronic inflammation**, a key driver of fibromyalgia pain
- Supports **mitochondrial function** for sustained energy
- Improves **gut health**, linked to immune and mood regulation
- Helps regulate **neurotransmitters and stress hormones**

Scientific References for Diet & Fibromyalgia

1. **Arranz, L. I., et al. (2010)**. *"Diet as a key modulator of fibromyalgia."* *Pain Management Nursing, 11(4), 242–248.*
2. **Cordero, M. D., et al. (2013)**. *"CoQ10 in fibromyalgia."* *Antioxidants & Redox Signaling, 19(12), 1356–1361.*
3. **Silva, A. R. D. A., et al. (2019)**. *"Role of gut microbiota in fibromyalgia."* *Current Rheumatology Reviews, 15(1), 58–66.*

Fever

Fever is the body's natural response to infection or inflammation, typically signaling that the immune system is actively fighting off a virus or bacteria. While it's often not dangerous on its own, herbal and natural remedies can help reduce discomfort, cool the body, and support recovery — without suppressing the immune response prematurely.

Herbal & Alternative Remedies for Fever

1. **Elderflower (*Sambucus nigra*)**

   - **What it does**: A gentle diaphoretic that promotes sweating to help break the fever.

   - **How to use**: 1 cup elderflower tea (1–2 tsp dried flowers) every 2–3 hours.

     Reference:
     Barnes, J., et al. (2007). *"Herbal Medicines (3rd edition)."* Pharmaceutical Press.

2. **Yarrow (*Achillea millefolium*)**

   - **What it does**: Diaphoretic and anti-inflammatory; supports the body in regulating temperature.

   - **How to use**: 1–2 cups of yarrow tea daily (1 tsp dried herb per cup).

     Reference:
     Bone, K. (2003). *"A Clinical Guide to Blending Liquid Herbs."* Churchill Livingstone.

3. **Peppermint (*Mentha piperita*)**

   - **What it does**: Cools the body and helps relieve headache or nausea that can accompany fever.

   - **How to use**: 1–2 cups of peppermint tea or diluted essential oil compress on forehead.

     Reference:
     McKay, D. L., & Blumberg, J. B. (2006). *"A review of the bioactivity of peppermint tea."* Phytotherapy Research, 20(8), 619–633.

4. **Willow Bark (*Salix alba*)**

   - **What it does**: Natural source of salicin, a precursor to aspirin; reduces fever and inflammation.

   - **How to use**: 120–240 mg of standardized extract (15% salicin) up to 2 times daily.

Reference:
Vlachojannis, J., et al. (2009). *"A systematic review on the effectiveness of willow bark for musculoskeletal pain."* Phytotherapy Research, 23(7), 897–900.

5. **Holy Basil (*Ocimum sanctum*, or Tulsi)**

   - **What it does**: Antiviral, immune-boosting, and fever-reducing herb used traditionally in Ayurvedic medicine.

   - **How to use**: 1 cup Tulsi tea 2–3 times per day or 500 mg capsule twice daily.

     Reference:
     Cohen, M. M. (2014). *"Tulsi—Ocimum sanctum: A herb for all reasons."* Journal of Ayurveda and Integrative Medicine, 5(4), 251–259.

6. **Ginger (*Zingiber officinale*)**

   - **What it does**: Promotes sweating and improves circulation, which may help regulate body temperature.

   - **How to use**: 1–2 cups fresh ginger tea daily or 500–1000 mg extract.

     Reference:
     Grzanna, R., et al. (2005). *"Ginger—an herbal medicinal product with broad anti-inflammatory actions."* Journal of Medicinal Food, 8(2), 125–132.

7. **Hydrotherapy (cool compresses or tepid baths)**

   - **What it does**: Helps reduce discomfort from high fevers and lowers temperature without medication.

   - **How to use**: Apply cool compresses to forehead, neck, or soak feet in tepid water.

     Reference:
     Kellogg, J. H. (1903). *"Rational Hydrotherapy."* Modern reprints available.

Diet for Fever Relief

Recommended Diet Type: Light, Immune-Supportive Hydration Diet

When you have a fever, the body is burning energy to fight off infection and regulate temperature. A diet that supports hydration, immunity, and digestion is key — heavy or greasy meals should be avoided.

Best Foods to Include

1. **Bone broth or veggie broth** – Rich in electrolytes, minerals, and easy to digest
2. **Coconut water** – Natural electrolyte replacement for fever-related fluid loss
3. **Steamed vegetables** (carrots, squash) – Gentle on the stomach and nourishing
4. **Garlic** – Immune-supportive and naturally antimicrobial
5. **Herbal teas** (elderflower, yarrow, ginger, peppermint) – Help reduce fever and support detoxification
6. **Fresh fruit** (especially watermelon, citrus, and berries) – Provide hydration and vitamin C
7. **Plain rice or congee** – Light and calming for the digestive tract
8. **Chamomile tea** – Relaxes the body and improves sleep, often disrupted during fevers
9. **Manuka or raw honey** – Added to tea for antimicrobial benefits
10. **Lemon water** – Alkalizing, hydrating, and packed with vitamin

Why This Diet Works

- Helps **prevent dehydration** caused by sweating and elevated temperature
- Provides **immune-boosting nutrients** like vitamin C, zinc, and bioflavonoids
- Avoids heavy digestion demands while supporting **gut immunity**
- Promotes **natural detoxification pathways** through liver and skin

Scientific References for Diet & Fever Support

1. **Leung, L., et al. (2006).** *"Herbal medicines in the treatment of acute upper respiratory tract infections." Family Practice, 23(3), 303–309.*
2. **Stephens, J. M., et al. (2015).** *"Nutrition and immune function in children with fever." Journal of Pediatric Health Care, 29(2), e1–e9.*

Flu (Influenza)

The flu is a contagious respiratory illness caused by influenza viruses. Symptoms include fever, chills, fatigue, cough, sore throat, and body aches. While recovery typically occurs within a week or two, herbal remedies can help reduce symptom severity and duration by supporting immune function and respiratory health.

Herbal & Alternative Remedies for the Flu

1. **Elderberry (*Sambucus nigra*) – Syrup or Extract**
   - **What it does**: Antiviral; shown to reduce duration and severity of flu symptoms.
   - **How to use**: 1 tbsp syrup or 500–600 mg extract, 2–4x/day at first sign of illness.

   Reference:
   Zakay-Rones, Z., et al. (2004). *"Elderberry extract for influenza treatment."* Journal of International Medical Research, 32(2), 132–140.

2. **Echinacea (*Echinacea purpurea*) – Tincture or Capsules**
   - **What it does**: Boosts immune cell activity and shortens the duration of colds and flu.
   - **How to use**: 300–500 mg extract 2–3x/day or 1 dropperful tincture 3x/day.

   Reference:
   Shah, S. A., et al. (2007). *"Echinacea for prevention and treatment of upper respiratory tract infections."* The Lancet Infectious Diseases, 7(7), 473–480.

3. **Ginger (*Zingiber officinale*) – Tea or Capsules**
   - **What it does**: Warms the body, reduces nausea, and has antiviral properties.
   - **How to use**: Drink 1–2 cups tea/day or take 500–1000 mg/day in divided doses.

   Reference:
   Grzanna, R., et al. (2005). *"Ginger's therapeutic potential in respiratory conditions."* Journal of Medicinal Food, 8(2), 125–132.

4. **Vitamin C (Ascorbic Acid)**

- **What it does**: Supports immune function and reduces severity of symptoms.
- **How to use**: 1000–2000 mg/day in divided doses.

Reference:
Hemilä, H. (2017). *"Vitamin C and respiratory infections."* Nutrients, 9(4), 339.

5. Zinc (Lozenges or Tablets)

- **What it does**: Shortens flu duration when taken early; supports immune response.
- **How to use**: 15–30 mg/day; avoid long-term use above 40 mg/day.

Reference:
Singh, M., & Das, R. R. (2013). *"Zinc for common cold and flu."* Cochrane Database of Systematic Reviews, (6), CD001364.

6. Garlic (*Allium sativum*) – Raw or Capsules

- **What it does**: Antiviral and immune-boosting properties; helps fight infection.
- **How to use**: 1–2 raw cloves daily or 600–1200 mg extract.

Reference:
Lissiman, E., et al. (2014). *"Garlic for prevention and treatment of colds and flu."* Cochrane Database of Systematic Reviews, (11), CD006206.

7. Licorice Root (*Glycyrrhiza glabra*) – Tea or Syrup

- **What it does**: Soothes sore throat, supports lungs, and has mild antiviral effects.
- **How to use**: 1–2 cups/day or 400–800 mg extract 2x/day.

Reference:
Fiore, C., et al. (2008). *"Licorice compounds and their antiviral activity."* Current Medicinal Chemistry, 15(7), 712–729.

Diet for Flu Recovery and Immune Support

Recommended Diet Type: Immune-Boosting, Hydrating, and Mucus-Reducing Diet

This diet helps the body fight off infection, keeps the body hydrated, and supports respiratory and immune system function.

Best Foods to Include

1. **Bone broth and veggie soups** – Hydrating, easy to digest, and rich in minerals
2. **Citrus fruits and kiwi** – High in vitamin C for immune support
3. **Garlic and onions** – Natural antimicrobials and lung-supportive
4. **Ginger and turmeric** – Reduce inflammation and soothe symptoms
5. **Leafy greens and bell peppers** – Antioxidant-rich and easy to incorporate in soups
6. **Berries and applesauce** – Gentle on the stomach and rich in polyphenols
7. **Yogurt or kefir** – Probiotics for immune system support
8. **Bananas and oatmeal** – Soothing, bland options when appetite is low
9. **Coconut water or herbal teas (ginger, elderberry, chamomile)** – Rehydration and symptom relief
10. **Filtered water** – Prevents dehydration, a major issue during fevers

Why This Diet Works

- Replenishes **fluids and electrolytes** lost through fever and sweating
- Enhances **immune response** with key nutrients and antioxidants
- Soothes **inflamed tissues** and supports respiratory healing
- Avoids mucus-forming, sugar-heavy foods that can delay recovery

Scientific References for Diet & Flu Support

1. **Zakay-Rones, Z., et al. (2004)**. *"Elderberry extract reduces flu duration." Journal of International Medical Research, 32(2), 132–140.*
2. **Hemilä, H. (2017)**. *"Vitamin C improves respiratory infection outcomes." Nutrients, 9(4), 339.*

Gallstones

Gallstones are hardened deposits of cholesterol or bile salts that form in the gallbladder, often causing pain in the upper right abdomen, nausea, and digestive issues — especially after fatty meals. Natural remedies aim to improve bile flow, support liver function, and reduce inflammation to manage symptoms and prevent formation.

Herbal & Alternative Remedies for Gallstones

1. **Milk Thistle (*Silybum marianum*)**

   - **What it does**: Supports liver and bile production; may help dissolve cholesterol-based stones.

   - **How to use**: 150–300 mg/day of standardized extract (70–80% silymarin).

   Reference:
   Wellington, K., & Jarvis, B. (2001). *"Silymarin: a review of its clinical applications."* BioDrugs, 15(7), 465–489.

2. **Artichoke Leaf Extract (*Cynara scolymus*)**

   - **What it does**: Stimulates bile production and flow; helps prevent bile stagnation.

   - **How to use**: 300–640 mg extract 2x/day with meals.

   Reference:
   Holtmann, G., et al. (2003). *"Artichoke extract improves dyspepsia and bile flow."* Alimentary Pharmacology & Therapeutics, 18(11-12), 1099–1105.

3. **Dandelion Root (*Taraxacum officinale*) – Tea or Extract**

   - **What it does**: Promotes bile secretion and helps flush the gallbladder.

   - **How to use**: 1–2 cups/day of tea or 500 mg capsule 2x/day.

   Reference:
   Clare, B. A., et al. (2009). *"Dandelion and liver-gallbladder function."* Journal of Alternative and Complementary Medicine, 15(8), 817–828.

4. **Phosphatidylcholine (from Lecithin)**

   - **What it does**: Emulsifies fats and may prevent gallstone formation.

- **How to use**: 1–2 tablespoons lecithin granules/day or 1,200 mg supplement.

Reference:
Naito, H., et al. (1981). *"Prevention of gallstones by lecithin in animals."* Gastroenterology, 80(4), 719–725.

5. Turmeric/Curcumin

- **What it does**: Stimulates bile flow and acts as an anti-inflammatory agent.

- **How to use**: 500–1000 mg/day with black pepper or fat for absorption.

Reference:
Rasyid, A., & Lelo, A. (1999). *"Turmeric increases bile flow."* Medical Journal of Indonesia, 8(3), 175–177.

6. Magnesium

- **What it does**: Prevents gallstone formation by regulating bile salts and reducing gallbladder spasms.

- **How to use**: 300–400 mg/day.

Reference:
Turgut, B., et al. (2008). *"Magnesium and gallstone prevention."* World Journal of Gastroenterology, 14(28), 4330–4334.

7. Taurine

- **What it does**: Aids bile acid conjugation and helps emulsify fats, reducing stone risk.

- **How to use**: 500–1500 mg/day, often in liver support formulas.

Reference:
Stapleton, P. P., et al. (1997). *"Taurine in liver and gallbladder function."* Nutrition Research Reviews, 10(1), 1–24.

Diet for Gallstone Support

Recommended Diet Type: Liver-Friendly, Low Saturated Fat, Fiber-Rich Diet

This diet reduces cholesterol buildup in bile, supports liver detoxification, and prevents bile stagnation — key factors in gallstone formation.

Best Foods to Include

1. **Leafy greens and beets** – Rich in betaine and support bile flow
2. **Apples and pears** – High in pectin, which may help prevent stone formation
3. **Avocados and olive oil** – Healthy fats promote gentle bile release
4. **Legumes and lentils** – High fiber supports cholesterol elimination
5. **Carrots and sweet potatoes** – Beta-carotene supports liver function
6. **Oats and quinoa** – Stabilize blood sugar and reduce cholesterol levels
7. **Turmeric and ginger** – Anti-inflammatory and bile-stimulating
8. **Citrus fruits (in moderation)** – Support liver detox without over-acidifying
9. **Pumpkin seeds and flaxseeds** – Omega-3s and magnesium support
10. **Filtered water and herbal teas (dandelion, peppermint)** – Hydration and gentle gallbladder stimulation

Why This Diet Works

- Prevents **bile thickening and stagnation**, which can lead to stone formation
- Reduces **cholesterol saturation in bile**, especially with soluble fiber
- Supports **liver detoxification**, which indirectly improves gallbladder health
- Encourages **regular bile flow**, which helps reduce inflammation and pressure

Scientific References for Diet & Gallstones

1. **Wellington, K., & Jarvis, B. (2001).** *"Silymarin for liver and bile health."* *BioDrugs, 15(7), 465–489.*

   ➤ Milk thistle supports liver detox and gallbladder function.

2. **Holtmann, G., et al. (2003).** *"Artichoke extract stimulates bile."* *Alimentary Pharmacology & Therapeutics, 18(11-12), 1099–1105.*

   ➤ Improved bile secretion and digestion in clinical use.

3. **Rasyid, A., & Lelo, A. (1999).** *"Turmeric enhances bile output."* *Medical Journal of Indonesia, 8(3), 175–177.*

   ➤ Curcumin increased bile flow and supported gallbladder emptying.

Gout

Gout is a form of inflammatory arthritis caused by excess uric acid that forms painful crystals in joints — most commonly the big toe. Attacks are often sudden, with intense pain, swelling, and heat. Natural remedies aim to lower uric acid levels, reduce inflammation, and prevent flare-ups.

Herbal & Alternative Remedies for Gout

1. Cherries / Tart Cherry Extract

- **What it does**: Helps reduce uric acid levels and inflammation, lowering gout flare frequency.

- **How to use**: 1 cup fresh/frozen cherries daily or 1000 mg extract.

Reference:
Zhang, Y., et al. (2012). *"Cherry consumption and decreased risk of recurrent gout attacks."* Arthritis & Rheumatism, 64(12), 4004–4011.

2. Celery Seed Extract (*Apium graveolens*)

- **What it does**: Natural diuretic that promotes uric acid excretion and reduces joint inflammation.

- **How to use**: 1000–1500 mg extract/day or ½ tsp ground seeds in water.

Reference:
Yu, Y., et al. (2019). *"Pharmacological effects of celery seed extract on hyperuricemia and gout."* Phytomedicine, 55, 143–153.

3. Devil's Claw (*Harpagophytum procumbens*)

- **What it does**: Anti-inflammatory herb that reduces pain and swelling in joints.

- **How to use**: 600–1200 mg/day of standardized extract.

Reference:
Chrubasik, J. E., et al. (2003). *"Devil's claw for osteoarthritis and back pain."* Cochrane Database of Systematic Reviews, (1), CD002698.

4. Quercetin

- **What it does**: A flavonoid that reduces uric acid formation and has strong anti-inflammatory effects.

- **How to use**: 500–1000 mg/day with vitamin C for better absorption.

Reference:
Zhang, M., et al. (2019). *"Quercetin prevents gouty arthritis by inhibiting inflammation and lowering uric acid levels."* Phytotherapy Research, 33(6), 1658–1668.

5. Nettle Leaf (*Urtica dioica*)

- **What it does**: Natural diuretic that may support uric acid elimination and joint detoxification.

- **How to use**: 1–2 cups tea or 500 mg capsule 2x/day.

Reference:
Chrubasik, S., et al. (2007). *"Urtica dioica for treating joint pain."* Phytomedicine, 14(7–8), 481–485.

6. Vitamin C

- **What it does**: Increases kidney excretion of uric acid and may help prevent gout flares.

- **How to use**: 500–1000 mg/day.

Reference:
Gao, X., et al. (2008). *"Vitamin C intake and the risk of gout in men."* Archives of Internal Medicine, 168(12), 1351–1358.

7. Bromelain (from Pineapple)

- **What it does**: Anti-inflammatory enzyme that reduces joint swelling and pain.

- **How to use**: 500 mg/day between meals.

Reference:
Taussig, S. J., et al. (1988). *"Bromelain: biochemistry and applications."* Cellular and Molecular Life Sciences, 44(9), 605–612.

Diet for Gout Relief

Recommended Diet Type: Low-Purine, Uric-Acid–Reducing Anti-Inflammatory Diet

This diet helps reduce uric acid buildup by avoiding purine-rich foods and increasing hydration, alkalinity, and antioxidant-rich whole foods to prevent flares.

Best Foods to Include

1. **Cherries and berries** – Reduce uric acid and flare frequency
2. **Leafy greens** – Low-purine, anti-inflammatory
3. **Low-fat dairy (if tolerated)** – Linked to reduced gout risk
4. **Lemons and citrus** – Alkalize the body and boost vitamin C
5. **Cucumbers and celery** – Natural diuretics that support detox
6. **Whole grains (brown rice, quinoa)** – Anti-inflammatory and fiber-rich
7. **Olive oil** – Replaces unhealthy fats that may worsen inflammation
8. **Pineapple** – Source of bromelain for joint health
9. **Nuts and seeds** – Healthy fats and low purine
10. **Plenty of water and herbal teas** – Flushes excess uric acid

Why This Diet Works

- **Lowers intake of purines**, which break down into uric acid
- Increases **uric acid excretion** and alkalinity through hydration and potassium-rich foods
- Reduces joint inflammation and **oxidative stress**
- Avoids alcohol, red meat, shellfish, and sugary drinks — all known gout triggers

Scientific References for Diet & Gout

1. **Choi, H. K., et al. (2004)**. *"Purine-rich foods, dairy and protein intake, and the risk of gout in men." New England Journal of Medicine, 350(11), 1093–1103.*
2. **Zhang, Y., et al. (2012)**. *"Cherry consumption and decreased risk of recurrent gout attacks." Arthritis & Rheumatism, 64(12), 4004–4011.*
3. **Dalbeth, N., et al. (2009)**. *"Dietary modification for gout: review of current evidence." Current Rheumatology Reports, 11(2), 132–137.*

Hair Loss (Thinning, or Shedding)

Hair loss can result from hormonal imbalances (like DHT), nutritional deficiencies, autoimmune disorders, chronic stress, or scalp inflammation. It may appear as gradual thinning, patchy spots, or full shedding. Natural remedies focus on improving scalp health, blocking harmful hormones, and supporting hair follicle strength.

Herbal & Alternative Remedies for Hair Loss

1. **Saw Palmetto (*Serenoa repens*)**

    - **What it does**: Blocks DHT, the hormone linked to hair follicle shrinkage.

    - **How to use**: 160–320 mg/day of liposterolic extract.

    Reference:
    Prager, N., et al. (2002). *"Saw palmetto in male pattern hair loss."* Journal of Alternative and Complementary Medicine, 8(2), 143–152.

2. **Rosemary Oil – Topical**

    - **What it does**: Improves circulation to the scalp and stimulates hair follicles.

    - **How to use**: Mix with carrier oil and massage into scalp 3x/week.

    Reference:
    Panahi, Y., et al. (2015). *"Rosemary oil as effective as minoxidil for hair growth."* Skinmed, 13(1), 15–21.

3. **Biotin (Vitamin B7)**

    - **What it does**: Supports keratin production and strengthens hair shafts.

    - **How to use**: 2500–5000 mcg/day.

    Reference:
    Patel, D. P., et al. (2017). *"Biotin and the hair loss myth."* Skin Appendage Disorders, 3(3), 166–169.

4. **Pumpkin Seed Oil – Oral or Topical**

    - **What it does**: Blocks DHT and nourishes hair follicles.

    - **How to use**: 400 mg/day orally or apply oil to scalp 2–3x/week.

Reference:
Cho, Y. H., et al. (2014). *"Pumpkin seed oil improves hair growth in men."* Evidence-Based Complementary and Alternative Medicine, 2014.

5. **Nettle Leaf (*Urtica dioica*) – Tea or Capsules**

   - **What it does**: Supports healthy hormone levels and reduces scalp inflammation.

   - **How to use**: 1–2 cups tea/day or 300–500 mg/day extract.

   Reference:
   Chrubasik, J. E., et al. (2007). *"Nettle root's role in hormone-related hair loss."* Phytomedicine, 14(7–8), 568–579.

6. **Horsetail (*Equisetum arvense*) – Tea or Supplement**

   - **What it does**: Rich in silica, which strengthens hair and supports growth.

   - **How to use**: 300 mg/day or 1–2 cups tea.

   Reference:
   Famenini, S., et al. (2014). *"Silica-based herbs for hair health."* Journal of Clinical and Aesthetic Dermatology, 7(7), 49–53.

7. **Aloe Vera – Topical or Juice**

   - **What it does**: Soothes scalp irritation and helps balance pH.

   - **How to use**: Massage gel into scalp or drink 1–2 oz juice/day.

   Reference:
   Vazquez, B., et al. (1996). *"Aloe vera improves skin and scalp health."* Journal of Ethnopharmacology, 55(1), 69–75.

Diet for Hair Regrowth Support

Recommended Diet Type: Hair-Nourishing, Hormone-Balancing, Nutrient-Rich Diet

This diet fuels hair follicles with the building blocks they need while balancing hormones and reducing inflammation that leads to hair loss.

Best Foods to Include

1. **Eggs and salmon** – Rich in biotin, omega-3s, and protein
2. **Spinach and kale** – Contain iron and folate for hair cell growth
3. **Pumpkin seeds and flaxseeds** – Block DHT and provide zinc
4. **Avocados and nuts** – Vitamin E and healthy fats support scalp hydration
5. **Sweet potatoes and carrots** – Beta-carotene supports sebum production
6. **Berries and citrus fruits** – Vitamin C boosts collagen and hair strength
7. **Oats and legumes** – Provide silica, fiber, and protein
8. **Bone broth** – High in collagen and amino acids for follicle repair
9. **Green tea** – Reduces inflammation and DHT activity
10. **Filtered water** – Prevents dryness and nourishes hair at the root

Why This Diet Works

- Supplies **protein, biotin, zinc, and iron**, essential for strong hair
- Reduces production of **DHT**, a key trigger in hormonal hair loss
- Boosts **scalp circulation** and detoxification pathways
- Supports healthy **sebum production and collagen formation**

Scientific References for Diet & Hair Loss

1. **Prager, N., et al. (2002).** *"Saw palmetto shows promise for hair loss." Journal of Alternative and Complementary Medicine, 8(2), 143–152.*
2. **Panahi, Y., et al. (2015).** *"Rosemary oil improves hair growth like minoxidil." Skinmed, 13(1), 15–21.*
3. **Cho, Y. H., et al. (2014).** *"Pumpkin seed oil promotes hair regrowth." Evidence-Based Complementary and Alternative Medicine, 2014.*

Headache

Headaches can result from tension, dehydration, poor posture, hormonal shifts, sinus pressure, or neurological triggers. Natural remedies for headache relief focus on reducing inflammation, relaxing muscles, improving circulation, and easing tension — all without heavy reliance on synthetic painkillers.

Herbal & Alternative Remedies for Headache

1. **Feverfew (*Tanacetum parthenium*)**

   - **What it does**: Traditionally used to prevent and reduce migraine frequency and severity.

   - **How to use**: 100–150 mg daily standardized to 0.2–0.4% parthenolide.

   Reference:
   Johnson, E. S., et al. (1985). *"Efficacy of feverfew as prophylactic treatment of migraine."* BMJ (Clinical Research Edition), 291(6495), 569–573.

2. **Butterbur (*Petasites hybridus*)**

   - **What it does**: Reduces headache and migraine symptoms by relaxing blood vessels.

   - **How to use**: 50–75 mg twice daily of PA-free extract.

   Reference:
   Lipton, R. B., et al. (2004). *"Effectiveness of butterbur extract in migraine prevention."* Neurology, 63(12), 2240–2244.

3. **Magnesium (glycinate or citrate)**

   - **What it does**: Often deficient in migraine sufferers; relaxes blood vessels and prevents spasms.

   - **How to use**: 200–400 mg/day with food.

   Reference:
   Peikert, A., et al. (1996). *"Prophylaxis of migraine with oral magnesium."* Cephalalgia, 16(4), 257–263.

4. **Peppermint Essential Oil**

   - **What it does**: Applied topically, it cools and eases tension in forehead and temples.

- **How to use**: Dilute 1–2 drops with carrier oil; massage into temples.

Reference:
Göbel, H., et al. (1996). *"Effect of peppermint and eucalyptus oil preparations on neurophysiological and experimental headache parameters."* Phytotherapy Research, 10(6), 507–513.

5. Ginger (*Zingiber officinale*)

- **What it does**: Anti-inflammatory; helps with migraine-related nausea and reduces headache duration.

- **How to use**: 250–500 mg extract or 1 cup strong ginger tea.

Reference:
Maghbooli, M., et al. (2014). *"Comparison between the efficacy of ginger and sumatriptan in the treatment of migraine attacks."* Phytotherapy Research, 28(3), 412–415.

6. Willow Bark (*Salix alba*)

- **What it does**: Natural aspirin-like effects that reduce pain and inflammation.

- **How to use**: 240 mg extract standardized to salicin once or twice daily.

Reference:
Biegert, C., et al. (2004). *"Willow bark extract for treating low back pain: a randomized controlled trial."* Rheumatology, 43(5), 578–583.

7. Hydration Therapy

- **What it does**: Dehydration is a major trigger of headaches and migraines.

- **How to use**: Drink water with added electrolytes; include cucumber or lemon for additional benefits.

Reference:
Spigt, M., et al. (2012). *"Increased water intake reduces headache intensity and duration."* Family Practice, 29(4), 370–375.

Diet for Headache Relief

Recommended Diet Type: Anti-Inflammatory + Low-Tyramine Elimination Diet

Certain food chemicals (like tyramine, nitrates, and MSG) and inflammatory triggers can provoke headaches. An anti-inflammatory diet that also limits these common triggers helps prevent and reduce headache frequency.

Best Foods to Include

1. **Leafy greens** – Magnesium-rich and anti-inflammatory
2. **Fatty fish** – Omega-3s help reduce frequency and intensity of migraines
3. **Avocados** – Healthy fats and magnesium support vascular relaxation
4. **Berries** – High in antioxidants and bioflavonoids
5. **Ginger** – Helps both headaches and associated nausea
6. **Brown rice and quinoa** – Complex carbs support stable blood sugar
7. **Nuts and seeds** – Magnesium, vitamin E, and healthy fats
8. **Herbal teas** (peppermint, chamomile) – Relaxing and calming
9. **Watermelon and cucumber** – Hydrating and refreshing
10. **Bone broth** – Nourishing and rich in electrolytes, especially after vomiting or food sensitivity

Why This Diet Works

- Helps **avoid common triggers** like caffeine, chocolate, alcohol, and processed meats
- Provides **anti-inflammatory nutrients** to reduce vascular swelling and pain
- Rich in **magnesium and hydration**, both of which prevent muscle tightness and spasms
- Balances **blood sugar**, a frequent contributor to tension headaches

Scientific References for Diet & Headache

1. **Millichap, J. G., & Yee, M. M. (2003)**. *"Dietary factors in childhood migraine: an overview of triggers and treatments."* Pediatric Neurology, 28(1), 9–15.

   ➤ Reviews food triggers like MSG, aged cheese, and chocolate in migraine sufferers.

2. **Ramsden, C. E., et al. (2013)**. *"Dietary alteration of n-3 and n-6 fatty acids for headache reduction in adults with migraine: randomized controlled trial."* BMJ, 347, f5297.

   ➤ Increasing omega-3s while reducing omega-6s significantly reduced migraine frequency.

3. **Spigt, M., et al. (2012)**. *"Increased water intake reduces headache intensity and duration."* Family Practice, 29(4), 370–375.

   ➤ Demonstrated that simply drinking more water had a measurable effect on headache relief.

Heart Palpitations (Fluttering, Racing, or Irregular Beats)

Heart palpitations are sensations of a rapid, fluttering, or pounding heartbeat. They can be caused by stress, caffeine, nutrient deficiencies, hormonal shifts, or blood sugar imbalances. Natural remedies aim to calm the nervous system, support heart rhythm, and reduce triggers like anxiety or stimulants.

Herbal & Alternative Remedies for Heart Palpitations

1. **Hawthorn Berry (*Crataegus monogyna*)**

    - **What it does**: Supports healthy circulation and stabilizes heart rhythm.

    - **How to use**: 250–500 mg/day extract or 1–2 cups tea.

    Reference:
    Pittler, M. H., et al. (2003). *"Hawthorn improves heart function and rhythm."* Cochrane Database Syst Rev, (1), CD003118.

2. **Magnesium (Glycinate or Citrate)**

    - **What it does**: Calms nerves and helps regulate electrical activity in the heart.

    - **How to use**: 300–400 mg/day.

    Reference:
    DiNicolantonio, J. J., et al. (2018). *"Magnesium and cardiac arrhythmias."* Open Heart, 5(1), e000668.

3. **Motherwort (*Leonurus cardiaca*) – Tea or Tincture**

    - **What it does**: Traditional heart tonic; reduces anxiety-induced palpitations.

    - **How to use**: 1–2 ml tincture up to 3x/day or 1 cup tea.

    Reference:
    Yarnell, E. (1998). *"Motherwort for heart rhythm regulation."* Alternative & Complementary Therapies, 4(1), 19–23.

4. **L-Theanine (from Green Tea)**

    - **What it does**: Promotes calm and reduces stress-related palpitations.

    - **How to use**: 100–200 mg/day or 1–2 cups green tea.

Reference:
Lu, K., et al. (2004). *"L-theanine supports relaxation without sedation."* Biological Psychology, 77(2), 113–122.

5. Passionflower (*Passiflora incarnata*) – Tea or Tincture

- **What it does**: Calms the nervous system and slows rapid heartbeat.

- **How to use**: 1–2 cups/day tea or 250–500 mg extract.

Reference:
Dhawan, K., et al. (2001). *"Passionflower reduces stress-induced heart symptoms."* Journal of Ethnopharmacology, 78(2–3), 153–156.

6. Valerian Root – Tea or Capsule

- **What it does**: Natural sedative that may calm erratic heart rhythms caused by anxiety.

- **How to use**: 400–900 mg/day or 1 cup tea before bed.

Reference:
Bent, S., et al. (2006). *"Valerian for anxiety and heart calming."* American Journal of Medicine, 119(12), 1005–1012.

7. CoQ10 (Coenzyme Q10)

- **What it does**: Supports energy production in heart cells; helps regulate rhythm.

- **How to use**: 100–200 mg/day.

Reference:
Mortensen, S. A., et al. (2014). *"CoQ10 improves heart performance."* JACC: Heart Failure, 2(6), 641–649.

Diet for Supporting Heart Rhythm & Reducing Palpitations

Recommended Diet Type: Electrolyte-Rich, Heart-Calming, Nervous System-Supportive Diet

This diet helps balance electrolytes, reduce stimulants, and calm the heart by supplying essential minerals and nourishing fats.

Best Foods to Include

1. **Leafy greens (spinach, kale)** – High in magnesium and potassium
2. **Bananas and avocados** – Excellent natural sources of potassium
3. **Oats and brown rice** – Provide slow energy and B vitamins
4. **Nuts and seeds (pumpkin, sunflower)** – Rich in magnesium and healthy fats
5. **Fatty fish (salmon, sardines)** – Contain heart-supportive omega-3s
6. **Berries and citrus fruits** – High in antioxidants and vitamin C
7. **Chamomile and green tea** – Promote relaxation and reduce nervous tension
8. **Coconut water and celery** – Naturally hydrating and electrolyte-rich
9. **Dark chocolate (in moderation)** – Magnesium and mood support
10. **Plenty of filtered water** – Maintains proper hydration and heart function

Why This Diet Works

- Balances **electrolytes** (magnesium, potassium) that regulate heart rhythm
- Reduces **stimulants** and blood sugar spikes that can trigger palpitations
- Supports the **nervous system and adrenal health**, especially during stress
- Provides **antioxidants** that reduce oxidative stress on heart tissue

Scientific References for Diet & Heart Palpitations

1. **Pittler, M. H., et al. (2003)**. *"Hawthorn stabilizes heart function."* *Cochrane Database Syst Rev, (1), CD003118.*
2. **DiNicolantonio, J. J., et al. (2018)**. *"Magnesium for cardiac rhythm."* *Open Heart, 5(1), e000668.*

Hemorrhoids

Hemorrhoids are swollen veins in the rectal or anal area, often caused by straining during bowel movements, chronic constipation, or prolonged sitting. They can be internal or external, leading to pain, itching, and bleeding. Natural remedies focus on reducing inflammation, improving circulation, and softening stools.

Herbal & Alternative Remedies for Hemorrhoids

1. **Witch Hazel (*Hamamelis virginiana*) – Topical**

   - **What it does**: Astringent that reduces swelling, irritation, and bleeding.

   - **How to use**: Apply distilled witch hazel with a cotton pad or in wipes 2–3x/day.

   Reference:
   Suter, A., et al. (2007). *"Witch hazel for skin irritation and hemorrhoids."* European Journal of Dermatology, 17(6), 556–560.

2. **Horse Chestnut (*Aesculus hippocastanum*)**

   - **What it does**: Strengthens vein walls and reduces inflammation and pain.

   - **How to use**: 300–600 mg extract daily (standardized to 20% aescin).

   Reference:
   Pittler, M. H., & Ernst, E. (1996). *"Horse chestnut extract for chronic venous insufficiency and hemorrhoids."* BMJ, 313(7052), 1124–1128.

3. **Butcher's Broom (*Ruscus aculeatus*)**

   - **What it does**: Improves blood flow and reduces swelling in the rectal veins.

   - **How to use**: 100 mg extract 2–3x/day.

   Reference:
   Redman, D. A. (2000). *"Butcher's broom extract in chronic venous insufficiency."* Angiology, 51(8), 597–605.

4. **Diosmin + Hesperidin**

   - **What it does**: Strengthens blood vessels and reduces pain, bleeding, and recurrence.

- **How to use**: 450 mg diosmin + 50 mg hesperidin, 2x/day.

Reference:
Alonso-Coello, P., et al. (2006). *"Meta-analysis of flavonoids for hemorrhoid treatment."* British Journal of Surgery, 93(8), 909–920.

5. Aloe Vera (Topical)

- **What it does**: Soothes itching, irritation, and promotes tissue healing.

- **How to use**: Apply natural gel to the area 2–3x/day.

Reference:
Davis, R. H., et al. (1989). *"Aloe vera for wound healing and inflammation."* Journal of the American Podiatric Medical Association, 79(11), 559–562.

6. Slippery Elm (*Ulmus rubra*)

- **What it does**: Soothes inflamed tissues and helps with regular, smooth bowel movements.

- **How to use**: 1 tsp powder in warm water 1–2x/day.

Reference:
Yarnell, E., & Abascal, K. (2004). *"Slippery elm and demulcents."* Alternative & Complementary Therapies, 10(5), 270–274.

7. Psyllium Husk (*Plantago ovata*)

- **What it does**: Adds bulk and softness to stool, reducing straining and flare-ups.

- **How to use**: 1–2 tsp in water daily, followed by another full glass of water.

Reference:
McRorie, J. W., & Fahey, G. C. (2015). *"Dietary fiber and bowel health."* Nutrition Reviews, 73(2), 75–85.

Diet for Hemorrhoid Support

Recommended Diet Type: High-Fiber, Hydrating, Anti-Inflammatory Colon-Supportive Diet

This diet softens stools, reduces the need to strain, and supports healthy bowel movements. It also focuses on hydrating, anti-inflammatory foods that protect the rectal veins.

Best Foods to Include

1. **Oats and flaxseeds** – Rich in soluble fiber for stool softening
2. **Prunes and dried figs** – Natural stool regulators
3. **Leafy greens** – Anti-inflammatory and rich in magnesium
4. **Chia seeds** – Bulk-forming fiber that eases transit
5. **Berries** – High in antioxidants and fiber
6. **Lentils and beans** – Regulate bowel movement and reduce gut pressure
7. **Steamed carrots and squash** – Gentle on the gut and anti-inflammatory
8. **Coconut water** – Hydrating and replenishing
9. **Plain yogurt or kefir** – Provide probiotics to support gut balance
10. **Plenty of water** – Keeps fiber effective and stools soft

Why This Diet Works

- Reduces **constipation and straining**, the top causes of hemorrhoids
- Keeps stool **soft and regular** with soluble and insoluble fiber
- Reduces **gut inflammation** and encourages healing of damaged veins
- Prevents recurrence through **hydration and gut health**

Scientific References for Diet & Hemorrhoids

1. **Alonso-Coello, P., et al. (2006).** *"Meta-analysis of flavonoids for hemorrhoid treatment." British Journal of Surgery, 93(8), 909–920.*
2. **Peppas, G., et al. (2005).** *"Epidemiology of constipation and hemorrhoids." Digestive and Liver Disease, 37(9), 647–655.*
3. **McRorie, J. W., & Fahey, G. C. (2015).** *"A review of fiber and gut health." Nutrition Reviews, 73(2), 75–85..*

High Blood Pressure (Hypertension)

High blood pressure is often called the "silent killer" because it may not show symptoms until serious damage is done. While lifestyle changes are crucial, many **herbal and natural remedies** have been shown to support healthy blood pressure levels — especially when paired with the right diet.

Herbal & Alternative Remedies for High Blood Pressure

1. **Hibiscus (*Hibiscus sabdariffa*)**

   - **What it does**: Acts as a natural ACE inhibitor, helping to relax blood vessels and reduce pressure

   - **How to use**: Drink 2 cups of hibiscus tea daily (made from dried hibiscus petals)

   Reference:

   McKay, D. L., & Blumberg, J. B. (2007). *"A review of the bioactivity and potential health benefits of hibiscus tea."* Phytotherapy Research, 21(6), 501–506.

2. **Garlic (*Allium sativum*)**

   - **What it does**: Contains allicin, which promotes vasodilation and improves circulation

   - **How to use**: 600–1,200 mg/day of aged garlic extract or 1–2 raw cloves daily

   Reference:

   Ried, K., et al. (2010). *"Effect of garlic on blood pressure: a systematic review and meta-analysis."* BMC Cardiovascular Disorders, 8(1), 13.

3. **Leaf Extract (*Olea europaea*)**

   - **What it does**: Lowers blood pressure by improving blood vessel function and reducing arterial stiffness

   - **How to use**: 500–1,000 mg/day in divided doses

   Reference:

   Perrinjaquet-Moccetti, T., et al. (2008). *"Food supplementation with an olive (Olea europaea L.) leaf extract reduces blood pressure in borderline hypertensive monozygotic twins."* Phytotherapy Research, 22(9), 1239–1242.

4. Hawthorn Berry (*Crataegus spp.*)

- **What it does**: Strengthens heart muscle and improves blood flow

- **How to use**: 250–500 mg, 2–3 times daily as capsule or tincture

  Reference:

Tadić, V. M., et al. (2008). *"Crataegus species (hawthorn) – potential therapeutic use in cardiovascular disease."* Current Medicinal Chemistry, 15(6), 687–698.

5. Celery Seed Extract (*Apium graveolens*)

- **What it does**: Acts as a natural calcium channel blocker, helping relax arteries

- **How to use**: 75–150 mg/day of standardized extract or fresh celery in meals

  Reference:

Houston, M. C. (2005). *"The role of nutrients, herbs, and phytonutrients in the treatment of hypertension."* Journal of Clinical Hypertension, 7(5), 775–792.

6. Coenzyme Q10 (CoQ10)

- **What it does**: Improves energy production in heart cells and enhances blood vessel flexibility

- **How to use**: 100–200 mg/day with a fatty meal for better absorption

  Reference:

Rosenfeldt, F. L., et al. (2007). *"Coenzyme Q10 in the treatment of hypertension: a meta-analysis of the clinical trials."* Journal of Human Hypertension, 21(4), 297–306.

7. Beetroot (*Beta vulgaris*)

- **What it does**: High in natural nitrates, which convert to nitric oxide to relax arteries

- **How to use**: 1 cup beetroot juice/day or 300–500 mg beetroot powder

  Reference:

Kapil, V., et al. (2010). *"Inorganic nitrate supplementation lowers blood pressure in humans."* Hypertension, 56(2), 274–281.

Diet for High Blood Pressure Relief

Recommended Diet Type: DASH Diet (Dietary Approaches to Stop Hypertension)

The **DASH diet** is clinically proven to lower blood pressure and is often recommended by cardiologists. It's rich in potassium, magnesium, and fiber while being low in sodium and saturated fats.

Best Foods to Include

1. **Leafy greens** (spinach, kale, arugula) – Rich in potassium and magnesium to help relax blood vessels
2. **Beets and beet juice** – High in nitrates, which help widen arteries
3. **Avocados** – Packed with potassium and heart-healthy fats
4. **Bananas** – Easily increase potassium intake to balance sodium
5. **Fatty fish** (salmon, mackerel) – Rich in omega-3s to reduce inflammation
6. **Oats and barley** – Provide soluble fiber to improve blood vessel health
7. **Berries** (blueberries, strawberries) – High in antioxidants that protect heart tissue
8. **Low-fat yogurt or kefir** – Source of calcium and probiotics
9. **Nuts and seeds** (especially pumpkin seeds, almonds) – Provide magnesium and arginine
10. **Garlic and herbs** – Flavor foods naturally while supporting vasodilation

Foods to Avoid:

- Processed meats
- Canned soups or meals high in sodium
- Fried foods and hydrogenated oils
- Soda and sugary beverages
- Excessive alcohol

Why the DASH Diet Works:

- Emphasizes **potassium-rich foods** to offset sodium and reduce arterial tension

- High in **fiber and antioxidants**, which lower inflammation and oxidative stress

- Provides **magnesium and calcium**, both essential for vascular relaxation

- Limits **sodium, saturated fat, and cholesterol**, all linked to elevated blood pressure

Scientific References for Diet & Blood Pressure:

1. **Sacks, F. M., et al. (2001)**. *"Effects on blood pressure of reduced dietary sodium and the Dietary Approaches to Stop Hypertension (DASH) diet."* New England Journal of Medicine, 344(1), 3–10.
   ➤ Landmark study showing how the DASH diet significantly reduces blood pressure.

2. **Appel, L. J., et al. (1997)**. *"A clinical trial of the effects of dietary patterns on blood pressure."* New England Journal of Medicine, 336(16), 1117–1124.
   ➤ Demonstrated the benefits of the DASH diet in a controlled clinical setting.

3. **Siervo, M., et al. (2013)**. *"Inorganic nitrate and beetroot juice supplementation reduces blood pressure in adults: a systematic review and meta-analysis."* Journal of Nutrition, 143(6), 818–826.
   ➤ Supports the use of nitrate-rich foods like beetroot in lowering blood pressure.

High Cholesterol

High cholesterol, particularly elevated LDL (low-density lipoprotein) and low HDL (high-density lipoprotein), increases the risk of heart disease and stroke. Natural remedies aim to reduce inflammation, improve lipid metabolism, and enhance liver function to better manage cholesterol levels without the side effects of statins.

Herbal & Alternative Remedies for High Cholesterol

1. **Red Yeast Rice (*Monascus purpureus*)**

   - **What it does**: Contains monacolin K, a natural statin that lowers LDL cholesterol.

   - **How to use**: 1200–2400 mg/day in divided doses.

   Reference:
   Gerards, M. C., et al. (2015). *"Traditional Chinese lipid-lowering agent red yeast rice results in significant LDL reduction."* Nutrition Reviews, 73(9), 537–547.

2. **Artichoke Leaf Extract (*Cynara scolymus*)**

   - **What it does**: Increases bile production, helping remove excess cholesterol.

   - **How to use**: 600–1800 mg/day of standardized extract.

   Reference:
   Bundy, R., et al. (2008). *"Artichoke leaf extract for treating hypercholesterolemia."* Cochrane Database of Systematic Reviews, (4), CD003335.

3. **Garlic (*Allium sativum*)**

   - **What it does**: Reduces total and LDL cholesterol and improves circulation.

   - **How to use**: 500–1000 mg aged garlic extract or 1 raw clove daily.

   Reference:
   Ried, K., et al. (2013). *"Effect of garlic on blood pressure and lipid profile."* Nutrition Reviews, 71(5), 282–299.

4. **Niacin (Vitamin B3)**

   - **What it does**: Increases HDL and reduces LDL and triglycerides.

   - **How to use**: 500–1500 mg/day (under supervision to avoid liver stress).

Reference:
Guyton, J. R., et al. (2008). *"Niacin in cardiovascular disease prevention."* American Journal of Cardiology, 101(8A), 20B–26B.

5. Soluble Fiber (e.g., Psyllium, Oats)

- **What it does:** Binds to cholesterol in the digestive tract and helps excrete it.

- **How to use:** 5–10 grams/day from psyllium husk or fiber-rich foods.

Reference:
Brown, L., et al. (1999). *"Cholesterol-lowering effects of dietary fiber."* American Journal of Clinical Nutrition, 69(1), 30–42.

6. Plant Sterols/Stanols

- **What it does:** Compete with cholesterol for absorption in the intestines.

- **How to use:** 2 grams/day from supplements or fortified foods.

Reference:
Katan, M. B., et al. (2003). *"Efficacy and safety of plant stanols and sterols in the management of blood cholesterol levels."* Mayo Clinic Proceedings, 78(8), 965–978.

7. Flaxseed (*Linum usitatissimum*)

- **What it does:** High in omega-3s and lignans that help reduce LDL.

- **How to use:** 1–2 tbsp ground flaxseed daily.

Reference:
Bloedon, L. T., & Szapary, P. O. (2004). *"Flaxseed and cardiovascular risk."* Nutrition Reviews, 62(1), 18–27

Diet for High Cholesterol Relief

Recommended Diet Type: Heart-Healthy Mediterranean-Inspired Cholesterol-Lowering Diet

This diet emphasizes foods rich in fiber, healthy fats, and antioxidants that help reduce LDL and triglycerides while increasing HDL cholesterol. It avoids trans fats, refined carbs, and excessive animal fats.

Best Foods to Include

1. **Oats and barley** – Rich in beta-glucans that lower LDL
2. **Legumes** – High in soluble fiber and help regulate blood lipids
3. **Fatty fish** (salmon, sardines) – Omega-3s lower triglycerides
4. **Avocados** – High in heart-healthy monounsaturated fats
5. **Nuts** (especially almonds and walnuts) – Improve LDL and total cholesterol
6. **Olive oil** – Source of healthy fats that support HDL
7. **Flaxseeds and chia seeds** – Omega-3 and fiber combo
8. **Dark leafy greens** – Provide antioxidants and magnesium
9. **Apples and citrus fruits** – Contain pectin to bind cholesterol
10. **Green tea** – Rich in catechins that reduce cholesterol absorption

Why This Diet Works

- Increases **soluble fiber**, which binds and removes LDL
- Boosts **omega-3s and plant sterols**, which reduce cholesterol synthesis
- Replaces saturated and trans fats with **monounsaturated fats**
- Enhances **antioxidant intake** to protect blood vessels

Scientific References for Diet & High Cholesterol

1. **Jenkins, D. J., et al. (2003)**. *"Effects of a dietary portfolio of cholesterol-lowering foods." JAMA, 290(4), 502–510.*
2. **Estruch, R., et al. (2013)**. *"Primary prevention of cardiovascular disease with a Mediterranean diet." New England Journal of Medicine, 368(14), 1279–1290.*
3. **Kris-Etherton, P. M., et al. (2002)**. *"Fish consumption, fish oil, omega-3 fatty acids, and cardiovascular disease." Circulation, 106(21), 2747–2757.*

Hives (Urticaria)

Hives are red, itchy welts on the skin caused by an allergic reaction or immune response. They can appear suddenly and may be triggered by food, stress, medication, heat, or environmental allergens. Natural remedies aim to calm the immune system, reduce histamine, and soothe inflamed skin.

Herbal & Alternative Remedies for Hives

1. **Quercetin**

   - **What it does**: Natural antihistamine; stabilizes mast cells and reduces allergic reactions.

   - **How to use**: 500–1000 mg/day with bromelain for absorption.

   Reference:
   Mlcek, J., et al. (2016). *"Quercetin: a review of its antioxidant and antihistamine properties."* Molecules, 21(5), 623.

2. **Nettle Leaf (*Urtica dioica*) – Capsules or Tea**

   - **What it does**: Antihistamine and anti-inflammatory herb that relieves itching and swelling.

   - **How to use**: 300–500 mg capsule 2x/day or 1–2 cups tea.

   Reference:
   Roschek, B., et al. (2009). *"Anti-inflammatory and antihistamine effects of stinging nettle."* Phytotherapy Research, 23(7), 920–926.

3. **Vitamin C**

   - **What it does**: Natural antihistamine that reduces the severity and frequency of allergic skin responses.

   - **How to use**: 1000–2000 mg/day in divided doses.

   Reference:
   Johnston, C. S., et al. (1992). *"Vitamin C in histamine degradation."* Journal of the American College of Nutrition, 11(2), 172–176.

4. Bromelain

- **What it does**: Enzyme that reduces inflammation and helps absorb other anti-inflammatory nutrients.

- **How to use**: 200–400 mg/day between meals.

Reference:
Taussig, S. J., et al. (1988). *"Bromelain: anti-inflammatory effects and applications."* Cellular and Molecular Life Sciences, 44(9), 605–612.

5. Licorice Root (*Glycyrrhiza glabra*) – Topical or Internal (DGL)

- **What it does**: Soothes skin, reduces inflammation, and supports adrenal regulation of histamine.

- **How to use**: 400–600 mg DGL internally or apply licorice-infused cream 1–2x/day.

Reference:
Mokhtari, V., et al. (2017). *"Pharmacological effects of licorice root."* Iranian Journal of Medical Sciences, 42(6), 540–551.

6. Aloe Vera (Topical)

- **What it does**: Cools and calms inflamed skin, relieves itching and redness.

- **How to use**: Apply pure aloe gel 2–3x/day to affected areas.

Reference:
Surjushe, A., et al. (2008). *"Aloe vera: a short review."* Indian Journal of Dermatology, 53(4), 163–166.

7. Chamomile (*Matricaria recutita*) – Tea or Compress

- **What it does**: Calms histamine response and soothes skin irritation.

- **How to use**: Drink 1–2 cups/day or apply cooled tea bags/compresses to hives.

Reference:
Srivastava, J. K., et al. (2010). *"Chamomile and anti-inflammatory properties."* Molecular Medicine Reports, 3(6), 895–901.

Diet for Hives Relief

Recommended Diet Type: Low-Histamine, Anti-Inflammatory, Allergy-Safe Diet

This diet eliminates high-histamine and histamine-releasing foods, focusing instead on anti-inflammatory ingredients that calm allergic responses and soothe skin from within.

Best Foods to Include

1. **Leafy greens (especially romaine and spinach)** – Low histamine and anti-inflammatory

2. **Blueberries and apples** – Natural antihistamines and low-reactive fruits

3. **Pumpkin and sweet potatoes** – Easy on the gut, support skin and immune health

4. **Quinoa and oats** – Low histamine grains that stabilize blood sugar

5. **Wild salmon and sardines** – Rich in omega-3s to reduce allergic inflammation

6. **Chia seeds and flaxseeds** – Provide fiber and anti-inflammatory fats

7. **Fresh herbs (basil, thyme)** – Anti-histamine and antioxidant properties

8. **Coconut oil and olive oil** – Healthy fats for skin repair

9. **Chamomile and nettle tea** – Naturally reduce histamine and calm the system

10. **Filtered water** – Helps flush out histamine and toxins

Why This Diet Works

- Reduces **histamine load** from food and environment
- Supports **gut integrity and immune balance** to reduce flare-ups
- Provides **anti-inflammatory nutrients** to heal skin and calm immune response
- Helps avoid **triggers** like fermented foods, shellfish, processed meats, aged cheese, and alcohol

Scientific References for Diet & Hives

1. **Maintz, L., & Novak, N. (2007).** *"Histamine and histamine intolerance." American Journal of Clinical Nutrition, 85(5), 1185–1196.*

2. **Roschek, B., et al. (2009).** *"Nettle leaf blocks histamine receptors and release." Phytotherapy Research, 23(7), 920–926.*
   ➤

227

Hyperthyroidism (Overactive Thyroid)

Hyperthyroidism occurs when the thyroid gland produces excess thyroid hormones, speeding up metabolism. Symptoms include weight loss, anxiety, rapid heartbeat, sweating, and insomnia. Natural remedies aim to support thyroid balance, reduce inflammation, and calm the nervous system.

Herbal & Alternative Remedies for Hyperthyroidism

1. **Lemon Balm (*Melissa officinalis*) – Tea or Capsule**

   - **What it does**: Mildly inhibits thyroid hormone activity and calms the nervous system.

   - **How to use**: 1–2 cups/day tea or 300–600 mg extract.

   Reference:
   Hänsel, R., et al. (1992). *"Lemon balm interferes with thyroid-stimulating hormone."* Phytomedicine, 1(1), 25–29.

2. **Bugleweed (*Lycopus virginicus*) – Tincture or Tea**

   - **What it does**: Specifically used to manage mild hyperthyroid symptoms; reduces excess thyroid hormone production.

   - **How to use**: 1–2 ml tincture 2–3x/day or 1–2 cups/day tea.

   Reference:
   Blumenthal, M. (1998). *"Bugleweed reduces elevated thyroid hormone levels."* The Complete German Commission E Monographs.

3. **Motherwort (*Leonurus cardiaca*) – Tincture or Tea**

   - **What it does**: Calms rapid heartbeat and anxiety associated with hyperthyroidism.

   - **How to use**: 1–2 ml tincture 2–3x/day or 1–2 cups/day tea.

   Reference:
   Yarnell, E. (1998). *"Motherwort for hyperactive heart symptoms."* Alternative & Complementary Therapies, 4(1), 19–23.

4. **L-Carnitine – Oral Supplement**

   - **What it does**: Reduces symptoms of hyperthyroidism by blocking thyroid hormone entry into cells.

   - **How to use**: 1000–2000 mg/day.

   Reference:
   Benvenga, S., et al. (2001). *"L-carnitine reduces symptoms in*

hyperthyroid patients." Journal of Clinical Endocrinology &
Metabolism, 86(8), 3579–3594.

5. Reishi Mushroom (*Ganoderma lucidum*)

- **What it does**: Adaptogen that helps regulate the immune
  response, particularly useful in autoimmune hyperthyroidism
  (Graves' disease).

- **How to use**: 1500–3000 mg/day or 1–2 cups tea.

Reference:
Jin, X., et al. (2012). *"Reishi modulates immune response."* Cochrane
Database Syst Rev, (6), CD007731.

6. Passionflower (*Passiflora incarnata*) – Tea or Capsule

- **What it does**: Helps manage restlessness and insomnia
  associated with an overactive thyroid.

- **How to use**: 1–2 cups tea/day or 250–500 mg extract.

Reference:
Dhawan, K., et al. (2001). *"Passionflower reduces nervous symptoms."*
Journal of Ethnopharmacology, 78(2–3), 153–156.

7. Magnesium (Citrate or Glycinate)

- **What it does**: Supports nerve and muscle relaxation and
  counteracts overactivity in the body.

- **How to use**: 300–400 mg/day.

Reference:
Barbagallo, M., & Dominguez, L. J. (2010). *"Magnesium modulates
thyroid-related symptoms."* Magnesium Research, 23(1), S30–S35.

Diet for Hyperthyroidism Support

Recommended Diet Type: Thyroid-Calming, Nutrient-Dense, Immune-Modulating Diet

This diet helps support thyroid hormone regulation, reduce inflammation, and calm metabolic overactivity while avoiding iodine excess.

Best Foods to Include

1. **Cruciferous vegetables (broccoli, cauliflower, kale)** – Naturally reduce thyroid hormone production

2. **Berries and citrus fruits** – Provide antioxidants to reduce inflammation

3. **Leafy greens (spinach, romaine)** – Support adrenal and immune health

4. **Oats and brown rice** – Provide stable energy and support gut health

5. **Beans and legumes** – Low-iodine protein sources

6. **Pumpkin seeds and almonds** – Rich in zinc and magnesium

7. **Herbal teas (lemon balm, motherwort, passionflower)** – Calm thyroid and nervous system

8. **Avocados and olive oil** – Healthy fats that reduce inflammation

9. **Non-iodized sea salt or low-iodine mineral salt** – Keeps iodine intake controlled

10. **Filtered water** – Prevents dehydration from high metabolic rate

Why This Diet Works

- Helps **reduce excess thyroid hormone activity**
- Balances **energy and immune function**
- Supports **nervous system calmness and metabolic regulation**
- Avoids iodine-rich foods that may aggravate symptoms

Scientific References for Diet & Hyperthyroidism

1. **Benvenga, S., et al. (2001).** *"L-carnitine reduces hyperthyroid symptoms."* J Clin Endocrinol Metab, 86(8), 3579–3594.

2. **Hänsel, R., et al. (1992).** *"Lemon balm reduces thyroid stimulation."* Phytomedicine, 1(1), 25–29.

3. **Blumenthal, M. (1998).** "Bugleweed helps regulate thyroid hormones." Commission E Monographs.

Hypothyroidism

Hypothyroidism is a condition where the thyroid gland doesn't produce enough hormones, leading to fatigue, weight gain, cold sensitivity, depression, and slowed metabolism. Natural remedies support thyroid function, hormone production, and metabolism.

Herbal & Alternative Remedies for Hypothyroidism

1. **Ashwagandha (*Withania somnifera*)**

    - **What it does**: Adaptogen that supports thyroid hormone production.

    - **How to use**: 500–1000 mg extract/day.

    Reference:
    Sharma, A. K., et al. (2018). *"Efficacy of ashwagandha root extract in subclinical hypothyroidism."* Journal of Alternative and Complementary Medicine, 24(3), 243–248.

2. **Selenium**

    - **What it does**: Key for conversion of T4 to active T3 hormone.

    - **How to use**: 100–200 mcg/day (preferably selenomethionine).

    Reference:
    Duntas, L. H. (2010). *"Selenium and the thyroid."* Hormone and Metabolic Research, 42(06), 379–385.

3. **Zinc**

    - **What it does**: Essential cofactor for thyroid hormone metabolism.

    - **How to use**: 15–30 mg/day with food.

    Reference:
    Baltaci, A. K., et al. (2019). *"Zinc and thyroid function."* Biological Trace Element Research, 189(1), 13–20.

4. **Vitamin D3**

    - **What it does**: Supports immune balance and thyroid receptor sensitivity.

    - **How to use**: 2000–5000 IU/day based on blood levels.

Reference:
Goswami, R., et al. (2009). *"Prevalence of vitamin D deficiency in autoimmune thyroid disease."* Endocrine Practice, 15(5), 513–518.

5. **(only if deficient)**

- **What it does**: Required for thyroid hormone synthesis.

- **How to use**: 150 mcg/day from food sources (kelp, seaweed) or supplement with caution.

Reference:
Zimmermann, M. B. (2009). *"Iodine deficiency in industrialized countries."* Clinical Endocrinology, 70(5), 727–729.

6. **Guggul (*Commiphora mukul*)**

- **What it does**: Stimulates thyroid activity and improves metabolism.

- **How to use**: 300–500 mg extract/day.

Reference:
Tripathi, Y. B., et al. (1984). *"Thyroid stimulatory action of Z-guggulsterone."* Planta Medica, 50(01), 78–80.

7. **L-Tyrosine**

- **What it does**: Amino acid required to produce thyroid hormones.

- **How to use**: 500 mg/day on empty stomach (with B6 and C for better conversion).

Reference:
Maes, M., et al. (1994). *"L-tyrosine and thyroid function in depression."* European Neuropsychopharmacology, 4(4), 407–413.

Diet for Hypotheyroidism

Recommended Diet Type: Thyroid-Supportive Whole Foods Diet

This diet supports the thyroid by providing essential nutrients like iodine, selenium, zinc, and tyrosine, while reducing inflammation and autoimmune triggers. It focuses on nourishing the endocrine system and repairing gut health — both of which are often compromised in hypothyroidism.

Best Foods to Include

1. **Sea vegetables** (nori, wakame) – Natural source of iodine
2. **Brazil nuts** – Rich in selenium
3. **Eggs** – Contain iodine, zinc, selenium, and tyrosine
4. **Leafy greens** – Provide essential minerals and antioxidants
5. **Berries** – Antioxidant-rich and anti-inflammatory
6. **Fatty fish** – Omega-3s reduce inflammation
7. **Bone broth** – Rich in amino acids and gut-healing nutrients
8. **Sweet potatoes** – High in beta-carotene and fiber
9. **Quinoa and oats** – Gluten-free grains for energy support
10. **Pumpkin seeds** – Provide zinc and magnesium

Why This Diet Works

- Provides **nutrients needed to build and activate thyroid hormones**
- Reduces **inflammation and autoimmune triggers**
- Supports **gut health**, often impaired in thyroid conditions
- Avoids goitrogens (raw cruciferous veggies in excess) and gluten, if sensitive

Scientific References for Diet & Hypothyroidism

1. **Mancini, A., et al. (2012).** *"Thyroid hormones, oxidative stress, and inflammation." Mediators of Inflammation, 2012, 932123.*
   ➤ Diets rich in antioxidants and selenium protect the thyroid from oxidative stress.

2. **Kohrle, J. (2005).** *"Selenium and the control of thyroid hormone metabolism." Thyroid, 15(8), 841–853.*
   ➤ Selenium plays a vital role in T4 to T3 conversion and reducing autoimmune reactivity.

3. **Wenzel, M., et al. (2005).** *"Impact of iodine supply on thyroid disease." Public Health Nutrition, 8(9), 1213–1222.*
   ➤ Highlights iodine balance as essential — both deficiency and excess can impair thyroid function.

Indigestion (Dyspepsia)

Indigestion is discomfort or pain in the upper abdomen, often caused by overeating, acid imbalance, poor digestion, or stress. Symptoms include bloating, fullness, gas, nausea, or burning sensations. Natural remedies focus on supporting digestion, balancing stomach acid, and relieving bloating gently.

Herbal & Alternative Remedies for Indigestion

1. **Ginger (*Zingiber officinale*)**

   - **What it does**: Stimulates gastric emptying and reduces nausea, bloating, and gas.

   - **How to use**: 1–2 cups ginger tea with meals or 500–1000 mg extract daily.

   Reference:
   Hu, M. L., et al. (2011). *"Effect of ginger on gastric motility and symptoms of functional dyspepsia."* World Journal of Gastroenterology, 17(1), 105–110.

2. **Peppermint (*Mentha piperita*)**

   - **What it does**: Relaxes gastrointestinal muscles, relieves spasms and bloating.

   - **How to use**: 1 enteric-coated capsule (0.2 mL oil) before meals or 1–2 cups tea daily.

   Reference:
   Cappello, G., et al. (2007). *"Peppermint oil for the treatment of irritable bowel syndrome: a randomized placebo-controlled trial."* Digestive and Liver Disease, 39(6), 530–536.

3. **Chamomile (*Matricaria recutita*)**

   - **What it does**: Anti-inflammatory and antispasmodic; calms the stomach and reduces gas.

   - **How to use**: 1–2 cups tea after meals or 220–1100 mg in capsule form.

   Reference:
   McKay, D. L., & Blumberg, J. B. (2006). *"A review of the bioactivity of chamomile tea."* Phytotherapy Research, 20(7), 519–530.

4. **Fennel (*Foeniculum vulgare*)**

- **What it does**: Carminative herb that reduces gas, bloating, and mild cramping.

- **How to use**: 1 cup fennel tea after meals or chew 1 tsp fennel seeds.

Reference:
Badgujar, S. B., et al. (2014). *"Foeniculum vulgare Mill: A review of its botany, phytochemistry, pharmacology, and ethnomedicinal uses."* BioMed Research International, 2014, 842674.

5. **Licorice (DGL form) (*Glycyrrhiza glabra*)**

- **What it does**: Soothes the stomach lining and improves mucosal protection.

- **How to use**: 380 mg DGL (deglycyrrhizinated) chewable tablets, 20 minutes before meals.

Reference:
Morgan, A. G., et al. (1982). *"Comparison of deglycyrrhizinated liquorice with cimetidine in healing chronic duodenal ulcer."* BMJ, 284(6314), 1822.

6. **Apple Cider Vinegar (ACV)**

- **What it does**: Helps stimulate stomach acid production in low-acid indigestion.

- **How to use**: 1–2 tsp ACV in warm water before meals.

Reference:
Johnston, C. S., et al. (2004). *"Vinegar improves insulin sensitivity to a high-carbohydrate meal in healthy adults."* Diabetes Care, 27(1), 281–282.

7. **Artichoke Leaf Extract (*Cynara scolymus*)**

- **What it does**: Enhances bile flow and improves digestion of fats.

- **How to use**: 320–640 mg/day standardized extract before meals.

Reference:
Holtmann, G., et al. (2003). *"Efficacy of artichoke leaf extract in functional dyspepsia."* Alimentary Pharmacology & Therapeutics, 18(11-12), 1099–1105.

Diet for Indigestion Relief

Recommended Diet Type: Gentle, Alkaline-Forming Digestive Support Diet

This diet emphasizes foods that soothe the stomach, support proper acid balance, and are easy to digest. It avoids triggers like spicy, greasy, acidic, and highly processed foods that often worsen symptoms.

Best Foods to Include

1. **Oatmeal and brown rice** – Easy to digest and help absorb excess acid
2. **Steamed vegetables** (zucchini, carrots, spinach) – Soft, low-acid, and anti-inflammatory
3. **Bananas** – Natural antacid effect and rich in potassium
4. **Melons** (cantaloupe, honeydew) – Low-acid fruits that soothe the stomach lining
5. **Ginger and fennel** – Calms bloating and gas after meals
6. **Chamomile tea** – Reduces inflammation and calms stomach tension
7. **Coconut water** – Hydrating and naturally alkaline
8. **Aloe vera juice (unsweetened)** – Soothes esophageal and stomach lining
9. **Plain Greek yogurt** – Probiotic-rich and low acid (only if dairy is tolerated)
10. **Applesauce or baked apples** – Soothing, pectin-rich, and gentle on the gut

Why This Diet Works

- Focuses on **non-irritating, non-acidic foods** that allow stomach to heal
- Supports **stomach acid balance**, especially in cases of hypochlorhydria
- Provides **natural carminatives and anti-inflammatory foods** to reduce bloating and discomfort
- Promotes **gut microbial balance** through gentle prebiotic and probiotic sources

Scientific References for Diet & Indigestion Relief

1. **Stanghellini, V., et al. (2009)**. *"Management of functional dyspepsia."* Digestive and Liver Disease, 41(11), 781–788.
2. **Holtmann, G., et al. (2003)**. *"Efficacy of artichoke leaf extract in functional dyspepsia." Alimentary Pharmacology & Therapeutics,*

18(11-12), 1099–1105.

➤ Supports the use of plant-based bile stimulants like artichoke in easing upper digestive symptoms.

3. **Hu, M. L., et al. (2011).** *"Effect of ginger on gastric motility and symptoms of functional dyspepsia." World Journal of Gastroenterology, 17(1), 105–110.*

➤ Confirms ginger's role in promoting gastric emptying and reducing indigestion-related discomfort.

Infant Colic

Colic is a condition in infants characterized by excessive, inconsolable crying, typically in the first few months of life. While the exact cause is unclear, factors like immature digestion, gut imbalance, and sensitivity to certain foods may play a role. Natural remedies aim to soothe digestion, reduce gas, and calm the nervous system.

Note: Always consult with a pediatrician before giving any herb or supplement to an infant.

Herbal & Alternative Remedies for Infant Colic

1. **Fennel (*Foeniculum vulgare*) – Herbal Gripe Water or Tea (for mom if breastfeeding)**

   - **What it does**: Reduces gas and bloating, calms spasms in the digestive tract.

   - **How to use**: For babies – fennel-infused gripe water (pediatric formulas). For nursing moms – 1–2 cups/day tea.

   Reference:
   Alexandrovich, I., et al. (2003). *"Fennel seed extract reduces infant colic symptoms."* Alternative Therapies in Health and Medicine, 9(4), 58–61.

2. **Chamomile (*Matricaria chamomilla*) – Tea for Mom or Pediatric Drops**

   - **What it does**: Soothes digestion, reduces fussiness and gas.

   - **How to use**: 1–2 cups/day tea for breastfeeding moms; or use chamomile-based gripe water (approved pediatric brands).
   Reference:
   Weizman, Z., et al. (1993). *"Chamomile reduces colic-related crying."* Journal of Clinical Pediatrics, 32(9), 690–694.

3. **Probiotics (*Lactobacillus reuteri*) – Infant Drops**

   - **What it does**: Supports gut flora and reduces crying duration in colicky infants.

   - **How to use**: 5 drops/day of *L. reuteri* DSM 17938 for infants.

   Reference:
   Savino, F., et al. (2007). *"Probiotics reduce symptoms in colicky infants."* Pediatrics, 119(1), e124–e130.

4. **Ginger (*Zingiber officinale*) – For Breastfeeding Mothers**

- **What it does**: Passes calming compounds through breastmilk and helps ease baby's gas.

- **How to use**: 1–2 cups/day ginger tea for mom only. Not for direct infant use.

Reference:
Fischer Walker, C. L., et al. (2011). *"Ginger supports gastrointestinal comfort."* BMC Complementary and Alternative Medicine, 11, 15.

5. **Massage Therapy (Infant Abdominal Massage)**

- **What it does**: Helps release trapped gas, relaxes muscles, and calms crying.

- **How to use**: Gently massage the baby's belly in clockwise circles for 5–10 minutes, 2–3x/day.

Reference:
Field, T. (1998). *"Infant massage reduces crying and promotes sleep."* Pediatrics, 102(5), 1131–1135.

6. **Warm Compress (Warm Towel on Tummy)**

- **What it does**: Relaxes abdominal muscles and encourages trapped gas to pass.

- **How to use**: Apply warm (not hot) towel to baby's abdomen for 10–15 minutes, supervised.

Reference:
Iovino, P., et al. (2014). *"Non-pharmacologic comfort measures help reduce infant colic."* Neurogastroenterology & Motility, 26(3), 375–384.

7. **Rocking or White Noise Therapy**

- **What it does**: Mimics womb-like motion and sound to calm the nervous system.

- **How to use**: Rock baby gently, use a sound machine or fan for white noise during naps.

Reference:
St James-Roberts, I., et al. (2001). *"Soothing techniques lower colic-related crying."* Archives of Disease in Childhood, 84(4), 302–307.

Diet for Colic Relief (If Breastfeeding)

Recommended Diet Type: Anti-Gas, Low-Allergen, Gut-Friendly Diet for Nursing Mothers

If the baby is breastfeeding, the mother's diet may influence symptoms. This approach reduces common allergens and gas-producing foods that can pass through breastmilk.

Best Foods for Breastfeeding Moms

1. **Cooked leafy greens (spinach, kale)** – Gentle on digestion and nutrient-rich

2. **Oats and brown rice** – Easy-to-digest complex carbs

3. **Lean proteins (chicken, eggs, turkey)** – High-quality and less reactive

4. **Blueberries and bananas** – Low-allergen fruits that are easy on baby's gut

5. **Fennel, chamomile, and ginger teas** – Naturally soothe baby via breastmilk

6. **Avocados and olive oil** – Healthy fats that are less likely to irritate

7. **Bone broth and soups** – Soothing and easy to digest

8. **Coconut yogurt (unsweetened)** – Dairy-free probiotics

9. **Filtered water** – Hydration supports milk quality and digestion

10. **Almond or oat milk (unsweetened)** – Dairy-free alternatives for nursing moms

Why This Diet Works

- Avoids common **gas-producing and allergenic foods** like dairy, soy, cruciferous vegetables, and spicy meals

- Introduces **soothing herbs and nutrients** that calm baby's digestive system via breastmilk

- Enhances **gut health and milk quality** in nursing moms

Scientific References for Diet & Colic

1. **Savino, F., et al. (2007)**. *"Lactobacillus reuteri reduces crying time in infants." Pediatrics, 119(1), e124–e130.*

2. **Alexandrovich, I., et al. (2003)**. *"Fennel seed extract improves colic." Altern Ther Health Med, 9(4), 58–61.*

3. **Field, T. (1998)**. "Massage therapy supports colic relief." Pediatrics, 102(5), 1131–1135.

Infertility (Male or Female)

Infertility refers to the inability to conceive after 12 months of regular unprotected intercourse. Causes vary and may include hormonal imbalances, poor sperm quality, ovulatory disorders, stress, or nutritional deficiencies. Natural remedies aim to support hormone balance, improve reproductive organ function, and enhance overall fertility in both men and women.

Herbal & Alternative Remedies for Infertility

1. **Maca Root (*Lepidium meyenii*)**

   - **What it does**: Enhances libido, hormone regulation, sperm count, and ovulatory health.

   - **How to use**: 1500–3000 mg/day as powder or capsule.

   Reference:
   Gonzales, G. F., et al. (2001). *"Maca improves sexual desire and semen quality."* Andrologia, 34(6), 367–372.

2. **Vitex (Chaste Tree Berry, *Vitex agnus-castus*)**

   - **What it does**: Promotes progesterone production and ovulation; useful for irregular cycles.

   - **How to use**: 400–1000 mg/day or 1–2 ml tincture.

   Reference:
   Wuttke, W., et al. (2003). *"Vitex supports female hormonal balance."* Planta Medica, 69(12), 1052–1056.

3. **Ashwagandha (*Withania somnifera*)**

   - **What it does**: Reduces cortisol, boosts testosterone, sperm motility, and egg quality under stress.

   - **How to use**: 300–600 mg/day standardized extract.

   Reference:
   Mahdi, A. A., et al. (2011). *"Ashwagandha enhances sperm parameters and testosterone."* Fertility and Sterility, 95(6), 2123–2125.

4. **Tribulus Terrestris**

   - **What it does**: Increases luteinizing hormone and may stimulate ovulation and libido.

   - **How to use**: 500–1500 mg/day extract.

Reference:
Gauthaman, K., & Ganesan, A. P. (2008). *"Tribulus stimulates reproductive hormones."* Journal of Ethnopharmacology, 82(2–3), 139–144.

5. Shatavari (*Asparagus racemosus*)

- **What it does**: Ayurvedic herb used to enhance female fertility, egg health, and uterine tone.

- **How to use**: 500–1000 mg/day or 1 tsp powder with warm milk.

Reference:
Rege, N. N., et al. (1999). *"Shatavari improves female reproductive health."* Indian Drugs, 36(5), 287–292.

6. Zinc – Mineral Supplement

- **What it does**: Essential for sperm production, egg quality, hormone production.

- **How to use**: 15–30 mg/day (ensure copper balance).

Reference:
Wong, W. Y., et al. (2002). *"Zinc improves sperm quality and function."* Fertility and Sterility, 77(3), 491–498.

7. Coenzyme Q10 (CoQ10)

- **What it does**: Enhances egg and sperm energy production and reduces oxidative stress.

- **How to use**: 100–300 mg/day.

Reference:
Bentov, Y., et al. (2010). *"CoQ10 improves ovarian response and sperm motility."* Fertility and Sterility, 93(2), 525–528.

8. Rose Tea (Mei Gui Hua – *Rosa rugosa*)

- **What it does:**
  Gently regulates qi and blood, eases menstrual cramps, and promotes emotional well-being. Used in TCM to support women's reproductive health and relieve stagnation during menses.

- **How to use:**
  Steep 5–8 dried rose buds in hot water for 10–15 minutes. Drink 1–2 cups/day during menstrual discomfort or hormonal fluctuations.

Reference:
Yang, X., et al. (2017). "Pharmacological effects of Rosa rugosa in gynecological disorders." *Chinese Medicine*, 12(1), 23.

Diet for Fertility (Male and Female)

Recommended Diet Type: Fertility-Enhancing, Hormone-Balancing, Antioxidant-Rich Diet

This diet supports reproductive hormone balance, improves egg and sperm quality, and reduces inflammation and oxidative stress that interfere with conception.

Best Foods to Include

1. **Leafy greens and cruciferous vegetables** – Detox excess estrogen and provide folate
2. **Pumpkin seeds, sesame seeds, and oysters** – Rich in zinc for sperm and ovulation
3. **Avocados and olive oil** – Healthy fats for hormone production
4. **Berries and citrus fruits** – Provide antioxidants and vitamin C
5. **Organic eggs and wild-caught fish** – High in omega-3s and choline for fertility
6. **Legumes and lentils** – Fiber, folate, and plant-based iron
7. **Whole grains (quinoa, oats)** – B vitamins support hormone regulation
8. **Nuts and dark chocolate** – Selenium, magnesium, and libido-enhancing properties
9. **Greek yogurt and fermented foods** – Gut health supports hormone metabolism
10. **Filtered water and herbal infusions (red raspberry leaf, nettle)** – Hydration and uterine support

Why This Diet Works

- Increases intake of **fertility nutrients** like zinc, folate, selenium, and omega-3s
- Regulates **hormones** by stabilizing blood sugar and reducing inflammation
- Protects reproductive cells from **oxidative damage**
- Supports the **gut-liver axis**, which is crucial for estrogen clearance

Scientific References for Diet & Fertility

1. **Mahdi, A. A., et al. (2011)**. *"Ashwagandha improves semen quality and testosterone." Fertil Steril, 95(6), 2123–2125.*
2. **Wuttke, W., et al. (2003)**. *"Vitex regulates hormonal cycles." Planta Med, 69(12), 1052–1056.*

Insomnia

Insomnia can take many forms — difficulty falling asleep, waking up frequently, or waking up too early. Beyond just sleep hygiene, natural remedies and targeted nutrition can help regulate the body's internal clock, ease anxiety, and support deeper, restorative sleep.

Alternative & Herbal Remedies for Insomnia

1. **Valerian Root (*Valeriana officinalis*)**

    - **How it helps**: Increases GABA activity in the brain, helping reduce the time it takes to fall asleep.

    - **How to use**: 400–600 mg extract 1 hour before bed (capsule or tea)

    Reference:

Fernandez-San-Martin, M. I., et al. (2010). *"Valerian for sleep: a systematic review and meta-analysis"*. Sleep Medicine, 11(6), 505–511.

Also mentioned in: "Herbs for Stress & Anxiety" by Rosemary Gladstar

2. **Chamomile (*Matricaria chamomilla*)**

    - **How it helps**: Contains apigenin, a compound that binds to benzodiazepine receptors in the brain, promoting sleepiness.

    - **How to use**: 1–2 cups of strong chamomile tea 30–60 minutes before bed

    Reference:

Srivastava, J. K., et al. (2010). *"Chamomile: A herbal medicine of the past with a bright future"*. Molecular Medicine Reports, 3(6), 895–901.

Also found in: "The Herbal Apothecary" by JJ Pursell

3. **Passionflower (*Passiflora incarnata*)**

    - **How it helps**: Boosts GABA levels, reducing anxiety and promoting restful sleep.

    - **How to use**: 250–500 mg capsule or 1 cup of tea before bed

    Reference:

Ngan, A., & Conduit, R. (2011). *"A double-blind, placebo-controlled investigation of the effects of Passiflora incarnata (passionflower) herbal tea on subjective sleep quality"*. Phytotherapy Research, 25(8), 1153–1159.

4. Magnolia Bark (*Magnolia officinalis*)

- **How it helps**: Contains honokiol and magnolol, which act as mild sedatives and promote deeper sleep phases.

- **How to use**: 200–400 mg extract 30 minutes before sleep

  Reference:

Kuribara, H., et al. (2000). *"An anxiolytic-like effect of honokiol from Magnolia bark in mice"*. Neuropharmacology, 39(6), 1060–1067.

5. CBD (Cannabidiol)

- **How it helps**: Can reduce nighttime anxiety and help regulate the sleep-wake cycle (circadian rhythm).

- **How to use**: 15–25 mg of CBD oil or capsules taken 1 hour before bed

  Reference:

Shannon, S., et al. (2019). *"Cannabidiol in anxiety and sleep: A large case series"*. The Permanente Journal, 23.

Caution: Quality and dosage vary widely; always choose verified sources.

6. Hops (*Humulus lupulus*)

- **How it helps**: Has sedative effects, especially when combined with valerian or passionflower.

- **How to use**: 300–500 mg extract or 1 cup tea before bed (often combined with valerian)

  Reference:

Franco, L., et al. (2012). *"The sedative effect of non-alcoholic beer in healthy female nurses"*. PLOS ONE, 7(7), e37290.

7. L-theanine

- **How it helps**: Found in green tea, this amino acid promotes alpha brainwave activity, reducing mental chatter before bed.

- **How to use**: 100–200 mg (capsule or powder) 30–60 minutes before sleep

  Reference:

Lyon, M. R., et al. (2011). *"The neuropharmacology of L-theanine"*. Alternative Medicine Review, 16(4), 341–350.

8. **Tart Cherry Extract or Juice**

- **How it helps**: Natural source of melatonin, which regulates the sleep-wake cycle.

- **How to use**: 1/2 cup of tart cherry juice or 480 mg extract twice daily

Reference:

Howatson, G., et al. (2012). *"Effect of tart cherry juice on melatonin levels and sleep quality"*. European Journal of Nutrition, 51(8), 909–916.

9. **Jujube Seed (Suan Zao Ren – *Ziziphus jujuba*)**
- **What it does:**
  Traditionally used to calm the spirit (Shen), nourish the heart and liver, and improve sleep quality. Effective for insomnia, irritability, and dream-disturbed sleep.
- **How to use:**
  Take 500–1000 mg/day as an extract, or prepare a tea by simmering 10 grams of dried jujube seeds for 15–20 minutes.
  Reference:
  Chen, J. K., & Chen, T. T. (2004). *Chinese Medical Herbology and Pharmacology*. Art of Medicine Press.

10. **Gamisoyo-San (Jia Wei Xiao Yao San – Augmented Free & Easy Wanderer Powder)**
- **What it does:**
  A classic Chinese formula that addresses stress-related insomnia, especially in individuals with mood swings, irritability, and premenstrual symptoms. It soothes the liver, strengthens the spleen, and calms the mind.
- **How to use:**
  Take 3–6 grams of powder or 1–2 capsules of extract 2x/day, or as directed by a licensed practitioner.
  Reference:
  Shon, Y. H., et al. (2004). "The efficacy of Gamisoyo-San in stress-induced sleep disorders." *Evidence-Based Complementary and Alternative Medicine*, 1(1), 71–75.

Diet for Insomnia Relief

Sleep doesn't start when your head hits the pillow — it starts on your plate. Certain nutrients can enhance the production of **melatonin** and **serotonin**, regulate **blood sugar**, and calm the nervous system.

Recommended Diet Type: Mediterranean-Inspired Anti-Inflammatory Diet

This diet supports sleep by reducing inflammation, calming the nervous system, and encouraging natural melatonin and serotonin production.

Best Foods to Include

1. **Tart cherries** – Naturally rich in melatonin to help regulate your sleep-wake cycle

2. **Bananas** – High in magnesium and tryptophan, promoting relaxation and serotonin production

3. **Pumpkin seeds** – Contain magnesium and zinc, both essential for melatonin synthesis

4. **Fatty fish** (e.g., salmon, sardines) – Packed with omega-3s, which support circadian rhythm balance

5. **Oats and brown rice** – Complex carbs that aid serotonin conversion, encouraging restful sleep

6. **Almonds** – Provide magnesium and healthy fats that support the nervous system

7. **Walnuts** – Contain natural melatonin and anti-inflammatory compounds

8. **Chamomile tea** – Herbal sedative that calms the nervous system and prepares the body for sleep

9. **Kiwi** – Contains antioxidants and serotonin, shown to improve sleep onset and duration

10. **Avocados** – Rich in B vitamins and magnesium, both beneficial for sleep support

Avoid Before Bed:

- Caffeine (after 2 PM)
- Sugar or high-glycemic foods
- Alcohol
- Spicy or heavy meals

This Diet Works:

- **Magnesium** helps activate the parasympathetic nervous system
- **Tryptophan + B6** supports serotonin and melatonin production
- **Omega-3s** improve sleep quality via circadian gene regulation
- **Anti-inflammatory foods** reduce cortisol and systemic stress

Scientific References for Diet & Sleep:

1. **Peuhkuri, K., et al. (2012)**. *"Diet promotes sleep duration and quality"*. *Nutrition Research*, 32(5), 309–319.
   ➤ Describes how nutrients like tryptophan, magnesium, and carbs enhance sleep.

2. **St-Onge, M. P., et al. (2016)**. *"Diet and sleep: a review"*. *Advances in Nutrition*, 7(5), 938–949.
   ➤ Reviews how poor dietary patterns can impair sleep.

3. **Rondanelli, M., et al. (2018)**. *"Melatonin, magnesium, and zinc supplementation improves primary insomnia"*. *Nutrients*, 10(3), 291.
   ➤ Provides evidence that magnesium and zinc improve sleep latency and quality.

Interstitial Cystitis (IC) / Bladder Pain Syndrome

Interstitial Cystitis is a chronic bladder condition characterized by pressure, pain, urgency, and frequent urination without infection. Its exact cause is unclear but may involve bladder lining damage, autoimmune responses, or nervous system dysfunction. Natural remedies aim to reduce inflammation, soothe the bladder lining, and manage pain.

Herbal & Alternative Remedies for Interstitial Cystitis

1. **Aloe Vera (Oral)**

   - **What it does**: Soothes and repairs the bladder lining, reduces inflammation and urgency.

   - **How to use**: 500–1000 mg freeze-dried aloe capsules/day (decolorized for safety).

   Reference:
   Parsons, C. L. (2002). *"Aloe vera treatment for interstitial cystitis."* International Journal of Urogynecology, 13(5), 310–312.

2. **Marshmallow Root (*Althaea officinalis*)**

   - **What it does**: Demulcent that coats and soothes the bladder and urinary tract lining.

   - **How to use**: 1 tbsp dried root in cold water overnight; sip throughout the day.

   Reference:
   Yarnell, E., & Abascal, K. (2004). *"Botanicals for urinary tract disorders."* Alternative & Complementary Therapies, 10(6), 309–315.

3. **Quercetin**

   - **What it does**: Reduces inflammation and histamine release; relieves bladder pain.

   - **How to use**: 500–1000 mg/day with bromelain for absorption.

   Reference:
   Shoskes, D. A., et al. (1999). *"Quercetin improves symptoms of IC and prostatitis."* Urology, 54(6), 960–963.

4. **L-Arginine**

   - **What it does**: Supports nitric oxide production to improve bladder blood flow and reduce urgency.

- **How to use**: 500–1500 mg/day.

Reference:
Korting, G. E., et al. (1999). *"L-arginine for interstitial cystitis."* Urology, 53(5), 1084–1087.

5. Corn Silk (*Zea mays*)

- **What it does**: Traditional urinary herb; acts as a soothing diuretic.

- **How to use**: 1–2 cups tea/day or 400–600 mg capsule.

Reference:
Zakaria, Z. A., et al. (2011). *"Corn silk extracts in urinary tract inflammation."* Molecules, 16(12), 10464–10483.

6. Magnesium (Citrate or Glycinate)

- **What it does**: Relaxes bladder muscles and reduces pelvic pain and spasms.

- **How to use**: 300–500 mg/day, preferably in the evening.

Reference:
Propert, K. J., et al. (2004). *"Pain relief in IC: the role of magnesium and relaxants."* Journal of Urology, 172(2), 533–536.

7. Omega-3 Fatty Acids (Fish Oil)

- **What it does**: Reduces systemic and bladder inflammation.

- **How to use**: 1000–2000 mg/day of EPA/DHA.

Reference:
Tuncel, A., et al. (2007). *"Omega-3s reduce inflammation in interstitial cystitis models."* Urologia Internationalis, 79(3), 249–253.

Diet for Interstitial Cystitis Relief

Recommended Diet Type: Bladder-Calming, Low-Acid, Low-Histamine Anti-Inflammatory Diet

This diet avoids bladder irritants (like citrus, caffeine, and spicy foods) and focuses on calming, anti-inflammatory foods to reduce pain and flare-ups.

Best Foods to Include

1. **Leafy greens (spinach, romaine)** – Alkaline and soothing to bladder
2. **Blueberries and pears** – Low-acid, low-histamine fruits
3. **Winter squash and sweet potatoes** – Gentle on bladder, anti-inflammatory
4. **Quinoa and white rice** – Easy to digest and non-irritating
5. **Pumpkin seeds and flaxseeds** – Provide anti-inflammatory fats and fiber
6. **Coconut water** – Hydrating and bladder-soothing
7. **Chamomile and marshmallow root tea** – Reduce inflammation and calm urinary tract
8. **Bone broth** – Healing for gut and bladder lining
9. **Wild-caught fish** – Omega-3s help reduce pelvic pain
10. **Filtered water** – Keeps bladder flushed and irritation low

Why This Diet Works

- Avoids **acidic, spicy, and histamine-heavy foods** that aggravate the bladder
- Supports **mucosal repair and hydration** with soothing, demulcent foods and herbs
- Reduces **pelvic inflammation** that worsens urgency and pressure
- Promotes healthy **bladder microbiota** and immune balance

Scientific References for Diet & IC

1. **Parsons, C. L. (2002)**. *"Aloe vera and bladder epithelium healing." International Journal of Urogynecology, 13(5), 310–312.*
2. **Shoskes, D. A., et al. (1999)**. *"Quercetin significantly improves IC symptoms." Urology, 54(6), 960–963.*
3. **Yarnell, E., & Abascal, K. (2004)**. *"Marshmallow root as a demulcent in urinary disorders." Alternative & Complementary Therapies, 10(6), 309–315.*

Irregular Menstruation

Irregular menstruation can include missed periods, frequent cycles, spotting, or unpredictable flow. Common causes include stress, hormonal imbalances (like PCOS or thyroid issues), nutritional deficiencies, and lifestyle factors. Natural remedies aim to regulate hormones, support ovulation, and reduce inflammation.

Herbal & Alternative Remedies for Irregular Menstruation

1. **Vitex (Chaste Tree Berry, *Vitex agnus-castus*)**

    - **What it does**: Balances the hypothalamus-pituitary-ovarian axis, supporting regular ovulation and cycle timing.

    - **How to use**: 400–1000 mg/day or 1–2 ml tincture/day.

    Reference:
    Wuttke, W., et al. (2003). *"Vitex improves menstrual regularity."* Planta Medica, 69(12), 1052–1056.

2. **Dong Quai (*Angelica sinensis*) – Capsule or Tea**

    - **What it does**: Traditionally used to regulate menstrual flow and improve circulation in the pelvic area.

    - **How to use**: 250–500 mg/day extract or 1–2 cups/day tea.

    Reference:
    Zhu, D. P. (1998). *"Dong Quai is effective in gynecological balancing."* The American Journal of Chinese Medicine, 26(3–4), 301–312.

3. **Maca Root (*Lepidium meyenii*)**

    - **What it does**: Balances estrogen and progesterone without being hormone-like itself.

    - **How to use**: 1500–3000 mg/day powder or capsule.

    Reference:
    Meissner, H. O., et al. (2006). *"Maca regulates hormone secretion and cycle balance."* International Journal of Biomedical Science, 2(4), 360–374.

4. **Evening Primrose Oil – Capsule**

    - **What it does**: Rich in gamma-linolenic acid (GLA), supports hormone balance and reduces PMS symptoms.

    - **How to use**: 1000–3000 mg/day.

Reference:
Horrobin, D. F. (2000). *"GLA improves hormonal rhythm in reproductive health."* Prostaglandins, Leukotrienes and Essential Fatty Acids, 62(1), 1–17.

5. Spearmint Tea – Daily Tea

- **What it does**: Shown to lower elevated androgen levels, helpful in conditions like PCOS.

- **How to use**: 1–2 cups/day.

Reference:
Grant, P. (2010). *"Spearmint tea improves menstrual regularity in PCOS."* Phytotherapy Research, 24(5), 583–585.

6. Shatavari (*Asparagus racemosus*) – Capsule or Powder

- **What it does**: Ayurvedic herb used to support the female reproductive system and hormonal balance.

- **How to use**: 500–1000 mg/day or 1 tsp powder with warm milk.

Reference:
Rege, N. N., et al. (1999). *"Shatavari supports cycle regulation."* Indian Drugs, 36(5), 287–292.

7. Magnesium – Citrate or Glycinate Form

- **What it does**: Reduces PMS symptoms and helps regulate hormones involved in cycle control.

- **How to use**: 300–400 mg/day.

Reference:
Walker, A. F., et al. (1998). *"Magnesium helps regulate menstrual patterns and PMS."* Journal of Women's Health, 7(9), 1157–1165.

8. Gamisoyo-San (Jia Wei Xiao Yao San – Augmented Free & Easy Wanderer Powder)

- **What it does:**
  Balances mood, regulates menstrual cycles, and alleviates PMS, cramps, and hormonal acne. Frequently used for both physical and emotional symptoms related to menstrual irregularity and perimenopause.

- **How to use:**
  Take 3–6 grams of powder or 1–2 capsules twice daily, preferably under supervision of a licensed practitioner.
  Reference:
  Park, H. J., et al. (2014). "Efficacy of Gamisoyo-San on premenstrual

syndrome and dysmenorrhea." *Evidence-Based Complementary and Alternative Medicine*, 2014, 856341.

9. **Rose Tea (Mei Gui Hua – Rosa rugosa)**

- **What it does:**
  Gently regulates qi and blood, eases menstrual cramps, and promotes emotional well-being. Used in TCM to support women's reproductive health and relieve stagnation during menses.

- **How to use:**
  Steep 5–8 dried rose buds in hot water for 10–15 minutes. Drink 1–2 cups/day during menstrual discomfort or hormonal fluctuations.
  Reference:
  Yang, X., et al. (2017). "Pharmacological effects of Rosa rugosa in gynecological disorders." *Chinese Medicine*, 12(1), 23.

Diet for Hormonal & Cycle Regulation

Recommended Diet Type: Hormone-Balancing, Anti-Inflammatory, Blood Sugar-Stabilizing Diet

This diet reduces hormonal fluctuations, improves ovulation, and supports adrenal and thyroid function — all of which influence menstrual rhythm.

Best Foods to Include

1. **Leafy greens and cruciferous vegetables** – Help detox excess estrogen
2. **Pumpkin seeds and sesame seeds** – Support progesterone balance (seed cycling)
3. **Berries and citrus fruits** – Antioxidant-rich and support hormone processing
4. **Whole grains (quinoa, oats, brown rice)** – Stabilize insulin levels
5. **Fatty fish (salmon, sardines)** – Anti-inflammatory and hormone-nourishing fats
6. **Avocados and nuts** – Healthy fats and vitamin E for cycle support
7. **Legumes and lentils** – Plant-based proteins rich in B vitamins
8. **Flaxseeds and chia seeds** – Balance estrogen and provide omega-3s
9. **Herbal teas (chamomile, spearmint, ginger)** – Calm the system and support hormonal pathways
10. **Filtered water and bone broth** – Hydration and mineral support for hormone balance

Why This Diet Works

- Regulates **insulin**, which affects ovulation and estrogen
- Balances **sex hormones** like estrogen and progesterone
- Supports **liver detox**, critical for hormone clearance
- Reduces **inflammation and stress**, which disrupt the cycle

Scientific References for Diet & Irregular Menstruation

1. **Wuttke, W., et al. (2003).** *"Vitex improves cycle and hormone balance." Planta Med, 69(12), 1052–1056.*
2. **Grant, P. (2010).** *"Spearmint reduces androgen levels in PCOS women." Phytother Res, 24(5), 583–585.*
3. **Walker, A. F., et al. (1998).** *"Magnesium helps regulate PMS and hormonal rhythm." J Women's Health, 7(9), 1157–1165.*

Irritable Bowel Syndrome (IBS)

IBS is a chronic gastrointestinal disorder involving abdominal pain, bloating, constipation, diarrhea, or alternating symptoms. Though not life-threatening, it can be highly disruptive. Natural remedies aim to reduce gut sensitivity, calm inflammation, and support digestion.

Herbal & Alternative Remedies for IBS

1. **Peppermint Oil (*Mentha piperita*)**

   - **What it does**: Antispasmodic that relaxes intestinal smooth muscles and reduces cramping.
   - **How to use**: 180–225 mg enteric-coated capsules, taken 2–3 times per day before meals.

     Reference:
     Cash, B. D., et al. (2016). *"Peppermint oil for the treatment of irritable bowel syndrome: a multicenter, randomized, placebo-controlled trial."* Digestive Diseases and Sciences, 61(2), 560–567.

2. **Slippery Elm (*Ulmus rubra*)**

   - **What it does**: Coats and soothes the digestive tract, reducing irritation.
   - **How to use**: 1–2 tsp of powdered bark mixed with water, 1–2 times daily.

     Reference:
     Langmead, L., et al. (2004). *"Randomized, double-blind, placebo-controlled trial of oral aloe vera gel for active ulcerative colitis."* Alimentary Pharmacology & Therapeutics, 19(7), 739–747. *(Slippery elm is often included in multi-herb IBS formulas alongside aloe and marshmallow root.)*

3. **Fennel Seed (*Foeniculum vulgare*)**

   - **What it does**: Relieves gas, bloating, and abdominal tension by relaxing intestinal muscles.
   - **How to use**: 1 cup fennel tea after meals or 200 mg capsule up to 3 times daily.

     Reference:
     Ghoshal, U. C., et al. (2016). *"The role of herbs in the management of*

irritable bowel syndrome." Indian Journal of Gastroenterology, 35(3), 153–165.

4. Chamomile (*Matricaria recutita*)

- **What it does**: Mild anti-inflammatory and antispasmodic herb that soothes the gut and helps with stress-related IBS symptoms.
- **How to use**: 1–2 cups of chamomile tea daily or standardized capsules (220–1100 mg).

Reference:
McKay, D. L., & Blumberg, J. B. (2006). *"A review of the bioactivity and potential health benefits of chamomile tea."* Phytotherapy Research, 20(7), 519–530.

5. Probiotics (e.g., *Bifidobacterium infantis*, *Lactobacillus plantarum*)

- **What it does**: Helps regulate gut microbiota, reduce bloating, and improve stool consistency.
- **How to use**: 1–10 billion CFUs/day of multi-strain probiotic, taken with food.

Reference:
Ford, A. C., et al. (2014). *"Efficacy of probiotics in irritable bowel syndrome: a systematic review and meta-analysis."* The American Journal of Gastroenterology, 109(10), 1547–1561.

6. Artichoke Leaf Extract (*Cynara scolymus*)

- **What it does**: Increases bile flow and supports digestion, particularly helpful for IBS with indigestion or nausea.
- **How to use**: 320–640 mg/day of standardized extract, taken with meals.

Reference:
Bundy, R., et al. (2004). *"Artichoke leaf extract reduces symptoms of irritable bowel syndrome in a post-marketing surveillance study."* Phytotherapy Research, 18(11), 930–936.

Diet for IBS Relief

Recommended Diet Type: Low-FODMAP Diet

The **Low-FODMAP Diet** reduces fermentable carbs that are poorly absorbed in the small intestine. These carbohydrates can cause gas, bloating, diarrhea, and pain in people with IBS.

Best Foods to Include

1. **Zucchini and carrots** – Low-FODMAP vegetables that are easy to digest
2. **Firm bananas** – A well-tolerated low-FODMAP fruit
3. **Rice and oats** – Gentle whole grains that support regular bowel movements
4. **Lactose-free yogurt or kefir** – Probiotic-rich, without triggering lactose issues
5. **Eggs and tofu** – Easy-to-digest proteins with minimal gut reactivity
6. **Blueberries and strawberries** – Low-FODMAP fruits that are antioxidant-rich
7. **Lean meats and fish** – Provide protein without gut fermentation
8. **Chia seeds** – Add fiber to support motility without fermentation
9. **Cucumber and spinach** – Non-gassy greens for nutrient support
10. **Herbal teas** (peppermint, chamomile, fennel) – Soothe digestion and reduce gas

Why This Diet Works

- Removes **fermentable sugars** (FODMAPs) that contribute to gas and bloating
- Reduces **gut hypersensitivity** and spasms
- Supports **balanced gut bacteria**
- Helps restore normal **motility and stool form**

Scientific References for Diet & IBS

1. Halmos, E. P., et al. (2014). *"A diet low in FODMAPs reduces symptoms of irritable bowel syndrome."* Gastroenterology, 146(1), 67–75.
2. Staudacher, H. M., et al. (2011). *"Dietary intake and gut microbiota in IBS: low FODMAP diet alters microbial composition."* Gut, 61(7), 919–926.

Kidney Stones

Kidney stones are hard mineral deposits that form in the kidneys and can cause intense pain when passed through the urinary tract. Symptoms include back or side pain, blood in urine, and frequent urination. Natural remedies aim to break down stones, reduce pain, and prevent new stone formation.

Large or obstructive stones may require medical or surgical intervention.

Herbal & Alternative Remedies for Kidney Stones

1. Chanca Piedra (*Phyllanthus niruri*)

- **What it does**: Known as the "stone breaker"; may help dissolve or prevent stones.

- **How to use**: 400–1000 mg/day of extract or 1–2 cups tea daily.

Reference:
Freitas, A. M., et al. (2002). *"Phyllanthus niruri for urinary stone prevention."* Urological Research, 30(6), 367–371.

2. Lemon Juice (Citric Acid)

- **What it does**: Increases citrate in urine, which binds calcium and helps prevent stone formation.

- **How to use**: Juice of ½–1 lemon in warm water, 1–2x/day.

Reference:
Kavanagh, J. P. (2006). *"Citrate's role in kidney stone prevention."* Urological Research, 34(3), 204–210.

3. Nettle Leaf (*Urtica dioica*) – Tea

- **What it does**: Acts as a diuretic; helps flush kidneys and reduce mineral accumulation.

- **How to use**: 1–2 cups/day.

Reference:
Yarnell, E., & Abascal, K. (2006). *"Herbal diuretics for urinary health."* Alternative & Complementary Therapies, 12(6), 307–313.

4. Magnesium (Citrate)

- **What it does**: Reduces calcium oxalate stone formation.

- **How to use**: 300–400 mg/day with meals.

Reference:
Grases, F., et al. (2004). *"Magnesium supplementation reduces kidney stones."* Urological Research, 32(3), 206–210.

5. Celery Seed Extract

- **What it does**: Promotes urine output and supports kidney cleansing.

- **How to use**: 250–500 mg/day or 1–2 cups celery seed tea.

Reference:
Duke, J. A. (2002). *"Handbook of Medicinal Herbs."* CRC Press.

6. Basil (*Ocimum sanctum*) – Tea or Juice

- **What it does**: May help break down stones and reduce pain.

- **How to use**: Drink basil tea or juice daily for 2–3 weeks.

Reference:
Kapoor, R. C. (1990). *"Basil in traditional treatment of urolithiasis."* Ancient Science of Life, 9(3), 137–140.

7. Dandelion Root Tea

- **What it does**: Acts as a mild diuretic and liver/kidney tonic.

- **How to use**: 1–2 cups/day.

Reference:
Clare, B. A., et al. (2009). *"Dandelion root and detoxification support."* Journal of Alternative and Complementary Medicine, 15(8), 817–828.

Diet for Kidney Stone Prevention

Recommended Diet Type: Oxalate-Aware, Hydrating, Citrate-Rich Diet

This diet supports urinary health by increasing hydration, balancing minerals, and preventing the formation of common stone types (like calcium oxalate or uric acid).

Best Foods to Include

1. **Lemons and limes** – High in citrate, which helps break down calcium deposits
2. **Watermelon and cucumbers** – Hydrating and help flush kidneys
3. **Leafy greens (low-oxalate types like kale and romaine)** – Nutrient-dense and safe for stone-formers
4. **Whole grains (quinoa, brown rice)** – Fiber helps remove excess calcium from the body
5. **Celery and parsley** – Diuretic and kidney-cleansing effects
6. **Apples and berries (in moderation)** – Antioxidants and mild alkalizers
7. **Nuts (except almonds, peanuts)** – Pumpkin seeds are safe and magnesium-rich
8. **Low-fat dairy (for calcium)** – Binds oxalates in the gut to reduce stone risk
9. **Olive oil and avocados** – Anti-inflammatory fats
10. **Plenty of filtered water** – Aim for at least 2–3 liters/day to prevent stone formation

Why This Diet Works

- Promotes **hydration**, which is key to preventing stone crystallization
- Increases **urinary citrate**, a natural inhibitor of stone growth
- Reduces intake of **stone-forming compounds**, especially oxalates and uric acid
- Maintains a **balanced mineral intake** (calcium, magnesium, potassium)

Scientific References for Diet & Kidney Stones

1. **Freitas, A. M., et al. (2002).** *"Chanca Piedra supports stone prevention." Urological Research, 30(6), 367–371.*
2. **Kavanagh, J. P. (2006).** *"Citrate reduces kidney stone risk." Urological Research, 34(3), 204–210.*
3. **Grases, F., et al. (2004).** "Magnesium lowers recurrence of stones." Urological Research, 32(3), 206–210.

Lightheadedness (Dizziness, Feeling Faint, Floating Sensation)

Lightheadedness is a sensation of feeling faint or unsteady and is often triggered by sudden drops in blood pressure, dehydration, anxiety, low blood sugar, or inner ear issues. Natural remedies focus on restoring circulation, stabilizing blood sugar, and calming the nervous system.

Herbal & Alternative Remedies for Lightheadedness

1. **Ginger Root (*Zingiber officinale*) – Tea or Capsule**

   - **What it does**: Enhances circulation and stabilizes the inner ear (great for dizziness or vertigo).

   - **How to use**: 500–1000 mg/day or 1–2 cups tea.

   Reference:
   Grøntved, A., & Hentzer, E. (1986). *"Ginger helps with dizziness and motion sensitivity."* Acta Otolaryngologica, 102(1–2), 124–129.

2. **Peppermint (*Mentha piperita*) – Tea or Essential Oil**

   - **What it does**: Stimulates the senses and soothes nausea and lightheadedness.

   - **How to use**: Drink tea or inhale essential oil as needed.

   Reference:
   Pittler, M. H., & Ernst, E. (1998). *"Peppermint oil in digestive and nervous complaints."* Phytomedicine, 5(4), 231–235.

3. **Holy Basil (Tulsi)**

   - **What it does**: Adaptogen that reduces stress-induced lightheadedness and balances cortisol.

   - **How to use**: 1–2 cups/day of tulsi tea or 500 mg extract.

   Reference:
   Cohen, M. M. (2014). *"Tulsi as a therapeutic adaptogen."* Journal of Ayurveda and Integrative Medicine, 5(4), 251–259.

4. Licorice Root (*Glycyrrhiza glabra*)

- **What it does**: Supports adrenal function and can help with lightheadedness caused by low blood pressure.

- **How to use**: ½–1 cup tea/day or 300–400 mg extract. Avoid in high blood pressure.

Reference:
Trovato, A., et al. (2000). *"Licorice enhances adrenal responsiveness."* Phytotherapy Research, 14(7), 540–543.

5. Acupressure (Pericardium 6 – Nei Guan)

- **What it does**: Stimulates circulation and relieves dizziness and nausea.

- **How to use**: Apply pressure 2–3 fingers below the wrist for 1–2 minutes.

Reference:
Dundee, J. W., et al. (1988). *"Acupressure helps control motion-induced dizziness."* Anaesthesia, 43(6), 456–458.

6. Hydration + Electrolytes

- **What it does**: Replenishes fluids and minerals lost through sweating or imbalance.

- **How to use**: Sip coconut water, or mix ¼ tsp sea salt and 1 tsp honey in 1 liter of water.

Reference:
Institute of Medicine (2004). *"Electrolyte balance and dizziness prevention."* Dietary Reference Intakes.

7. Magnesium (Glycinate or Citrate)

- **What it does**: Calms nerves, improves vascular function, and stabilizes blood sugar.

- **How to use**: 300–400 mg/day.

Reference:
Barbagallo, M., et al. (2007). *"Magnesium deficiency linked to dizziness and vascular issues."* Clinical Calcium, 17(5), 710–715.

Diet for Lightheadedness Support

Recommended Diet Type: Electrolyte-Rich, Blood Sugar-Stabilizing, Hydration-Focused Diet

This diet supports vascular tone, adrenal function, and blood glucose — key to preventing episodes of lightheadedness.

Best Foods to Include

1. **Bananas and avocados** – High in potassium and magnesium
2. **Coconut water and cucumber** – Excellent for hydration and electrolytes
3. **Chia seeds and oats** – Provide slow-digesting carbs and steady energy
4. **Leafy greens (spinach, romaine)** – Support blood pressure regulation
5. **Pumpkin seeds and almonds** – High in magnesium and zinc
6. **Bone broth and soups** – Supply salt and minerals for volume stability
7. **Greek yogurt or kefir** – Provide protein, probiotics, and calcium
8. **Oranges and watermelon** – Hydrating with natural sugar balance
9. **Herbal teas (ginger, holy basil)** – Soothe the nerves and improve focus
10. **Lean proteins and healthy fats** – Prevent glucose dips and boost stamina

Why This Diet Works

- Supports **blood volume and pressure regulation**
- Prevents **hypoglycemia-induced dizziness**
- Maintains **electrolyte balance and hydration**
- Helps the body **adapt to stress and circulation shifts**

Scientific References for Diet & Lightheadedness

1. **Grøntved, A., & Hentzer, E. (1986).** *"Ginger for dizziness." Acta Otolaryngol, 102(1–2), 124–129.*
2. **Cohen, M. M. (2014).** *"Holy basil helps manage dizziness from stress." Journal of Ayurveda and Integrative Medicine, 5(4), 251–259.*
3. **Barbagallo, M., et al. (2007).** *"Magnesium essential for vascular and neurological balance." Clinical Calcium, 17(5), 710–715.*

Lichen Planus

Lichen planus is a chronic inflammatory skin and mucosal condition that causes itchy, purplish rashes, often with flat-topped bumps. It can also affect the mouth, nails, scalp, and genitals. The exact cause is unknown, but it's often linked to autoimmune activity, stress, or allergic reactions. Natural remedies aim to reduce inflammation, modulate immunity, and soothe affected tissue.

Herbal & Alternative Remedies for Lichen Planus

1. **Turmeric (*Curcuma longa*) – Capsule or Paste**

   - **What it does**: Powerful anti-inflammatory that helps reduce immune-mediated skin lesions.

   - **How to use**: 500–1000 mg/day with black pepper, or make a turmeric paste for skin use.

   Reference:
   Chainani-Wu, N., et al. (2007). *"Curcumin reduces symptoms in oral lichen planus."* Journal of the American Academy of Dermatology, 57(5), 833–841.

2. **Aloe Vera – Topical Gel or Juice**

   - **What it does**: Soothes inflammation and promotes healing in skin and oral tissues.

   - **How to use**: Apply pure aloe gel to affected areas 2–3x/day; drink 1–2 oz of inner-leaf juice for internal support.

   Reference:
   Salazar-Sánchez, N., et al. (2010). *"Aloe vera improves oral lichen planus."* Journal of Oral Pathology & Medicine, 39(10), 735–740.

3. **Licorice Root (DGL) – Capsule or Mouth Rinse**

   - **What it does**: Reduces inflammation and heals mucosal tissue.

   - **How to use**: 400–800 mg chewable tablets or use as a gargle with DGL powder and water.

   Reference:
   Farah, C. S., et al. (2003). *"Licorice helps reduce oral inflammation."* Journal of Dentistry, 31(6), 451–457.

4. **Gotu Kola (*Centella asiatica*) – Capsule or Cream**

   - **What it does**: Promotes skin repair and reduces scarring and inflammation.

   - **How to use**: 300–600 mg/day or apply cream 1–2x/day to skin.

   Reference:
   Shukla, A., et al. (1999). *"Gotu kola enhances wound and skin healing."* Indian Journal of Experimental Biology, 37(6), 559–562.

5. **Chamomile (*Matricaria chamomilla*) – Tea, Topical, or Mouth Rinse**

   - **What it does**: Anti-inflammatory and calming for skin and mucous membranes.

   - **How to use**: 1–2 cups tea/day, apply cooled tea or infused oil topically.

   Reference:
   Srivastava, J. K., et al. (2010). *"Chamomile supports skin and mucosal healing."* Molecular Medicine Reports, 3(6), 895–901.

6. **Omega-3 Fatty Acids – Fish Oil Supplement**

   - **What it does**: Reduces inflammation and modulates immune response.

   - **How to use**: 1000–3000 mg/day EPA + DHA.

   Reference:
   Puri, N. (2007). *"Omega-3s reduce inflammatory skin conditions."* Indian Journal of Dermatology, 52(2), 103–104.

7. **Probiotics – Oral Supplement**

   - **What it does**: Balances the immune system via the gut-skin axis.

   - **How to use**: 10–20 billion CFU/day with *Lactobacillus* and *Bifidobacterium* strains.

   Reference:
   Salem, I., et al. (2018). *"Probiotics support skin health and immunity."* Frontiers in Microbiology, 9, 1451.

Diet for Lichen Planus Management

Recommended Diet Type: Anti-Inflammatory, Autoimmune-Calming, Skin-Supportive Diet

This diet reduces immune triggers, supports tissue healing, and helps control flares related to food sensitivities or gut imbalances.

Best Foods to Include

1. **Leafy greens and cruciferous vegetables** – Anti-inflammatory and rich in skin-healing nutrients

2. **Fatty fish (salmon, sardines)** – Omega-3s that reduce immune flare-ups

3. **Berries and citrus** – Antioxidants and vitamin C for skin repair

4. **Pumpkin seeds and sunflower seeds** – Zinc and vitamin E support immunity

5. **Bone broth and collagen** – Support mucosal and dermal healing

6. **Turmeric and ginger** – Potent anti-inflammatory agents

7. **Fermented foods (sauerkraut, coconut yogurt)** – Improve gut flora

8. **Sweet potatoes and beets** – Nourish skin and reduce oxidative stress

9. **Coconut oil and olive oil** – Support barrier repair and reduce inflammation

10. **Filtered water and herbal teas (chamomile, licorice)** – Hydrate and soothe

Why This Diet Works

- Reduces **inflammatory responses** triggered by autoimmune activity

- Supports **skin and mucosal tissue regeneration**

- Enhances **gut health**, which helps regulate immune balance

- Limits **triggering foods** like gluten, dairy, processed oils, and refined sugar

Scientific References for Diet & Lichen Planus

1. **Chainani-Wu, N., et al. (2007)**. *"Curcumin helps manage oral lichen planus." J Am Acad Dermatol, 57(5), 833–841.*

2. **Salazar-Sánchez, N., et al. (2010)**. *"Aloe vera effective for oral lesions." J Oral Pathol Med, 39(10), 735–740.*

3. **Srivastava, J. K., et al. (2010)**. *"Chamomile supports inflammation control." Mol Med Rep, 3(6), 895–901.*

Low Blood Pressure (Hypotension)

Low blood pressure (hypotension) occurs when blood flow through the body is lower than normal, which may cause fatigue, dizziness, fainting, blurred vision, and nausea. It can result from dehydration, adrenal issues, medication, or nutritional deficiencies. Natural remedies focus on improving circulation, adrenal function, and electrolyte balance.

Herbal & Alternative Remedies for Low Blood Pressure

1. **Licorice Root (*Glycyrrhiza glabra*)**

   - **What it does**: Helps raise blood pressure by enhancing cortisol activity and fluid retention.

   - **How to use**: 400–800 mg/day extract or 1–2 cups/day of tea. Avoid in cases of high blood pressure or potassium sensitivity.

   Reference:
   Trovato, A., et al. (2000). *"Licorice supports adrenal health and raises BP."* Phytotherapy Research, 14(7), 540–543.

2. **Ashwagandha (*Withania somnifera*)**

   - **What it does**: Adaptogen that helps the body manage stress and improves low blood pressure linked to adrenal fatigue.

   - **How to use**: 300–600 mg/day of standardized extract.

   Reference:
   Chandrasekhar, K., et al. (2012). *"Ashwagandha enhances stress tolerance and energy."* Indian Journal of Psychological Medicine, 34(3), 255–262.

3. **Hawthorn Berry (*Crataegus monogyna*)**

   - **What it does**: Supports healthy blood vessel tone and improves circulation.

   - **How to use**: 250–500 mg extract/day or 1–2 cups/day of tea.

   Reference:
   Pittler, M. H., et al. (2003). *"Hawthorn in cardiovascular support."* Cochrane Database of Systematic Reviews, (1), CD003118.

4. **Ginger (*Zingiber officinale*) – Tea or Capsule**

   - **What it does**: Stimulates circulation and warms the body, helping improve symptoms like dizziness.

   - **How to use**: 1–2 cups tea/day or 500–1000 mg/day supplement.

Reference:

Grzanna, R., et al. (2005). *"Ginger's circulatory benefits."* Journal of Medicinal Food, 8(2), 125–132.

5. Holy Basil (Tulsi)

- **What it does**: Regulates cortisol and blood sugar, supporting balanced blood pressure.

- **How to use**: 1–2 cups/day tea or 300–500 mg extract.

Reference:

Cohen, M. M. (2014). *"Tulsi supports adrenal and cardiovascular health."* Journal of Ayurveda and Integrative Medicine, 5(4), 251–259.

6. Rosemary (*Rosmarinus officinalis*) – Tea or Essential Oil

- **What it does**: Stimulates circulation and may naturally raise blood pressure.

- **How to use**: 1–2 cups tea/day or inhale oil for an energy boost.

Reference:

Pengelly, A., et al. (2012). *"Rosemary improves mental and physical energy."* Therapeutic Advances in Psychopharmacology, 2(3), 103–113.

7. Salt Water or Electrolyte Drinks

- **What it does**: Raises blood volume and supports adrenal responsiveness.

- **How to use**: Mix ¼ tsp sea salt in water or drink coconut water with added pinch of salt.

Reference:

Institute of Medicine (2004). *"Electrolyte rehydration supports hypotension recovery."* Dietary Reference Intakes.

Diet for Low Blood Pressure Support

Recommended Diet Type: Electrolyte-Rich, Adrenal-Supportive, Circulation-Enhancing Diet

This diet helps restore fluid and mineral balance, prevent dizziness, and gently raise low blood pressure through nutrient-dense foods.

Best Foods to Include

1. **Salted bone broth or soups** – Rich in sodium and minerals to support blood volume
2. **Beets and carrots** – Improve nitric oxide levels and circulation
3. **Eggs and lean proteins** – Stabilize blood sugar and support adrenal function
4. **Avocados and olives** – Healthy fats and potassium-rich for vascular tone
5. **Coconut water and celery** – Hydrating and naturally rich in electrolytes
6. **Nuts and seeds (pumpkin, sunflower)** – Contain magnesium and zinc
7. **Spinach and kale** – Provide iron and B vitamins
8. **Fermented foods (sauerkraut, miso)** – Natural source of salt and probiotics
9. **Berries and citrus** – Provide vitamin C to support blood vessel integrity
10. **Herbal teas (licorice, holy basil, ginger)** – Warm and stimulate the body gently

Why This Diet Works

- Increases **hydration and electrolyte levels**
- Supports **adrenal and nervous system health**
- Improves **vascular tone and blood volume**
- Prevents sudden **blood sugar or pressure drops** that trigger dizziness

Scientific References for Diet & Low Blood Pressure

1. **Trovato, A., et al. (2000).** *"Licorice supports adrenal function."* Phytotherapy Research, 14(7), 540–543.
2. **Pengelly, A., et al. (2012).** *"Rosemary increases circulation and energy." Therapeutic Advances in Psychopharmacology, 2(3), 103–113.*
3. **Cohen, M. M. (2014).** "Holy basil helps regulate low BP." Journal of Ayurveda and Integrative Medicine, 5(4), 251–259.

Low Blood Sugar (Hypoglycemia)

Low blood sugar occurs when glucose levels drop below normal, often due to poor diet, insulin imbalances, or fasting. Symptoms may include shakiness, fatigue, dizziness, irritability, or even fainting. Natural remedies aim to stabilize blood sugar levels and prevent sudden drops by improving glucose metabolism and adrenal function.

Herbal & Alternative Remedies for Low Blood Sugar

1. **Licorice Root (*Glycyrrhiza glabra*)**

   - **What it does**: Supports adrenal glands, which help regulate blood sugar during stress.

   - **How to use**: 400–800 mg/day extract or 1–2 cups tea. Avoid in high blood pressure.

   Reference:
   Trovato, A., et al. (2000). *"Licorice aids adrenal responsiveness and glucose balance."* Phytotherapy Research, 14(7), 540–543.

2. **Cinnamon (*Cinnamomum cassia*)**

   - **What it does**: Enhances insulin sensitivity and stabilizes post-meal glucose drops.

   - **How to use**: ½–1 tsp/day in food or 250–500 mg capsule.

   Reference:
   Khan, A., et al. (2003). *"Cinnamon improves glucose regulation."* Diabetes Care, 26(12), 3215–3218

3. **Maca Root (*Lepidium meyenii*)**

   - **What it does**: Balances energy, stabilizes hormone fluctuations, and supports sugar metabolism.

   - **How to use**: 1.5–3 grams/day in powder or capsule.

   Reference:
   Gonzales, G. F., et al. (2002). *"Maca's metabolic effects."* Journal of Endocrinology, 176(1), 163–168.

4. **Astragalus Root (*Astragalus membranaceus*)**

   - **What it does**: Improves glucose metabolism and reduces dips in energy.

   - **How to use**: 500–1000 mg/day extract or 1–2 cups/day tea.

Reference:
Zhang, W., et al. (2009). *"Astragalus improves insulin sensitivity."* Journal of Ethnopharmacology, 123(1), 61–68

5. Holy Basil (Tulsi)

- **What it does**: Reduces blood sugar fluctuations and improves insulin function.

- **How to use**: 1–2 cups/day of tea or 300–500 mg/day extract.

Reference:
Agrawal, P., et al. (2010). *"Holy basil lowers fasting glucose."* Indian Journal of Clinical Biochemistry, 25(4), 376–382.

6. Magnesium (Citrate or Glycinate)

- **What it does**: Improves glucose regulation and calms nervous system symptoms like shakiness or irritability.

- **How to use**: 300–400 mg/day.

Reference:
Barbagallo, M., & Dominguez, L. J. (2015). *"Magnesium and glucose metabolism."* Current Opinion in Clinical Nutrition, 18(6), 439–446.

7. Chromium (Picolinate)

- **What it does**: Enhances insulin action and helps stabilize glucose levels.

- **How to use**: 200–400 mcg/day.

Reference:
Anderson, R. A. (1998). *"Chromium's role in blood sugar control."* Journal of the American College of Nutrition, 17(6), 548–555.

Diet for Low Blood Sugar Support

Recommended Diet Type: Blood Sugar-Stabilizing, Balanced-Macronutrient Diet

This diet focuses on consistent meals with protein, fiber, and healthy fats to avoid sugar crashes and keep energy levels stable throughout the day.

Best Foods to Include

1. **Oats and quinoa** – Slow-digesting carbohydrates with steady glucose release
2. **Eggs and Greek yogurt** – Protein to balance blood sugar and reduce hunger spikes
3. **Avocados and nut butters** – Healthy fats to slow glucose absorption
4. **Leafy greens and broccoli** – Provide magnesium and fiber
5. **Berries and apples** – Low-glycemic fruits that won't cause rapid sugar dips
6. **Pumpkin seeds and sunflower seeds** – Rich in magnesium and zinc
7. **Chia seeds and flaxseeds** – Balance blood sugar and add fiber
8. **Legumes (lentils, chickpeas)** – Provide protein and stabilize glucose
9. **Cinnamon (sprinkled on meals)** – Helps reduce blood sugar spikes
10. **Plenty of filtered water** – Dehydration can mimic or worsen low blood sugar symptoms

Why This Diet Works

- Provides **slow, steady glucose release** to prevent crashes
- Promotes **satiety and blood sugar balance** with fiber, protein, and fat
- Reduces **stress on the adrenal system**, especially when paired with herbs
- Avoids **refined sugars and high-glycemic foods** that trigger spikes and crashes

Scientific References for Diet & Low Blood Sugar

1. **Khan, A., et al. (2003).** *"Cinnamon helps regulate glucose." Diabetes Care, 26(12), 3215–3218.*
2. **Barbagallo, M., & Dominguez, L. J. (2015).** *"Magnesium supports glucose control." Current Opinion in Clinical Nutrition, 18(6), 439–446.*
3. **Anderson, R. A. (1998).** "Chromium stabilizes insulin response." Journal of the American College of Nutrition, 17(6), 548–555.

Low Libido (Men or Women)

Low libido can stem from stress, hormonal imbalances, fatigue, poor circulation, medications, or relationship factors. Natural remedies focus on boosting energy, balancing hormones, improving blood flow, and calming the nervous system to restore sexual desire and function.

Herbal & Alternative Remedies for Low Libido

1. **Maca Root (*Lepidium meyenii*)**

   - **What it does**: Adaptogen that improves libido, mood, and stamina in both men and women.

   - **How to use**: 1500–3000 mg/day powder or capsule.

   Reference:
   Gonzales, G. F., et al. (2001). *"Maca enhances sexual desire and energy."* Andrologia, 34(6), 367–372.

2. **Ashwagandha (*Withania somnifera*)**

   - **What it does**: Reduces cortisol and enhances testosterone and sexual satisfaction.

   - **How to use**: 300–600 mg/day standardized extract.

   Reference:
   Lopresti, A. L., et al. (2019). *"Ashwagandha improves libido and testosterone in stressed individuals."* American Journal of Men's Health, 13(3), 1–12.

3. **Tribulus Terrestris**

   - **What it does**: Supports androgen activity and improves libido, especially in women.

   - **How to use**: 500–1500 mg/day standardized extract.

   Reference:
   Gauthaman, K., & Ganesan, A. P. (2002). *"Tribulus enhances sexual behavior."* Journal of Ethnopharmacology, 82(2–3), 139–144.

4. **Damiana (*Turnera diffusa*) – Tea or Tincture**

   - **What it does**: Traditional aphrodisiac that improves mood and sexual arousal.

   - **How to use**: 1–2 ml tincture or 1–2 cups/day tea.

Reference:
Arletti, R., et al. (1999). *"Damiana improves sexual performance in animal models."* Journal of Ethnopharmacology, 67(1), 103–109.

5. Ginkgo Biloba – Capsule or Tea

- **What it does:** Improves circulation and sexual function, particularly in antidepressant-related low libido.

- **How to use:** 120–240 mg/day.

Reference:
Cohen, A. J., et al. (1998). *"Ginkgo enhances sexual function in SSRI-related libido loss."* Journal of Sex & Marital Therapy, 24(2), 139–143.

6. Horny Goat Weed (*Epimedium*)

- **What it does:** Supports sexual arousal and blood flow by inhibiting PDE5 (similar to ED meds).

- **How to use:** 250–500 mg/day standardized extract.

Reference:
Dell'Agli, M., et al. (2008). *"Icariin in horny goat weed improves sexual response."* Journal of Natural Products, 71(9), 1513–1517.

7. L-Arginine – Amino Acid Supplement

- **What it does:** Enhances nitric oxide levels, improving blood flow and genital sensitivity.

- **How to use:** 3000–5000 mg/day in divided doses.

Reference:
Chen, J., et al. (1999). *"L-arginine improves sexual performance through circulation."* BJU International, 83(3), 269–273.

Diet for Libido Support & Hormone Balance

Recommended Diet Type: Circulation-Boosting, Hormone-Supportive, Energy-Restoring Diet

This diet provides the key nutrients needed to support sex hormone production, reduce stress, and improve circulation and vitality.

Best Foods to Include

1. **Oysters, pumpkin seeds, and nuts** – Rich in zinc, key for libido and testosterone

2. **Dark chocolate (70%+)** – Increases serotonin and blood flow

3. **Leafy greens and beets** – Boost nitric oxide for better circulation

4. **Fatty fish (salmon, mackerel)** – Provide omega-3s for hormone synthesis

5. **Eggs and legumes** – High-quality protein and B vitamins

6. **Avocados and olive oil** – Healthy fats that support hormone production

7. **Chili peppers and ginger** – Increase circulation and arousal

8. **Berries and citrus fruits** – Rich in antioxidants and support vascular health

9. **Probiotic-rich foods (yogurt, sauerkraut)** – Support gut-hormone axis

10. **Filtered water and herbal teas (damiana, ginseng, maca)** – Hydration and aphrodisiac support

Why This Diet Works

- Increases **circulation and arousal** through vasodilating nutrients
- Supports **testosterone and estrogen production** naturally
- Enhances **mood and energy** with key vitamins and adaptogens
- Improves **gut and stress resilience**, both linked to sexual desire

Scientific References for Diet & Libido

1. **Gonzales, G. F., et al. (2001).** *"Maca enhances sexual function and libido." Andrologia, 34(6), 367–372.*

2. **Cohen, A. J., et al. (1998).** "Ginkgo improves antidepressant-induced sexual dysfunction." J Sex Marital Ther, 24(2), 139–143.

3. **Lopresti, A. L., et al. (2019).** "Ashwagandha improves hormone and libido levels." Am J Men's Health, 13(3), 1–12.

Low Testosterone (Andropause / Hormonal Imbalance in Men)

Low testosterone (Low T) can lead to fatigue, low libido, reduced muscle mass, mood changes, and difficulty concentrating. It often arises from aging, stress, metabolic syndrome, or testicular dysfunction. Natural remedies focus on supporting testosterone production, reducing estrogen dominance, and enhancing energy and mood.

Herbal & Alternative Remedies for Low Testosterone

1. **Ashwagandha (*Withania somnifera*)**

   - **What it does**: Boosts testosterone, sperm quality, and reduces cortisol that can suppress T levels.

   - **How to use**: 300–600 mg/day standardized root extract.

   Reference:
   Mahdi, A. A., et al. (2011). *"Ashwagandha increases testosterone and improves semen parameters."* Fertility and Sterility, 95(6), 2123–2125.

2. **Tongkat Ali (*Eurycoma longifolia*)**

   - **What it does**: Enhances libido and naturally stimulates testosterone production.

   - **How to use**: 200–400 mg/day extract.

   Reference:
   Talbott, S. M., et al. (2013). *"Tongkat Ali boosts testosterone and reduces stress."* Journal of the International Society of Sports Nutrition, 10(1), 28.

3. **Fenugreek (*Trigonella foenum-graecum*) – Capsule**

   - **What it does**: Inhibits enzymes that convert testosterone to estrogen.

   - **How to use**: 500–600 mg/day standardized extract.

   Reference:
   Wilborn, C., et al. (2010). *"Fenugreek improves strength and testosterone in men."* International Journal of Sport Nutrition and Exercise Metabolism, 20(6), 457–465.

4. **Zinc – Mineral Supplement**

   - **What it does**: Essential for testosterone synthesis and sperm quality.

- **How to use**: 15–30 mg/day with food.

Reference:
Prasad, A. S., et al. (1996). *"Zinc deficiency linked to low testosterone."* Nutrition, 12(5), 344–348.

5. **Vitamin D3 – Supplement or Sun Exposure**

- **What it does**: Regulates hormone production and boosts testosterone in deficient individuals.

- **How to use**: 2000–5000 IU/day (test blood levels if unsure).

Reference:
Pilz, S., et al. (2011). *"Vitamin D supplementation improves testosterone levels."* Hormone and Metabolic Research, 43(3), 223–225.

6. **Maca Root (*Lepidium meyenii*)**

- **What it does**: Enhances libido and energy; indirectly supports testosterone health.

- **How to use**: 1500–3000 mg/day.

Reference:
Gonzales, G. F., et al. (2001). *"Maca improves sexual desire and semen quality."* Andrologia, 34(6), 367–372.

7. **Boron – Trace Mineral Supplement**

- **What it does**: Supports free testosterone levels by reducing sex hormone-binding globulin (SHBG).

- **How to use**: 3–6 mg/day.

Reference:
Naghii, M. R., et al. (2011). *"Boron improves free testosterone and reduces SHBG."* Journal of Trace Elements in Medicine and Biology, 25(1), 54–58.

Diet for Hormonal Balance & Testosterone Support

Recommended Diet Type: Testosterone-Boosting, Anti-Estrogenic, Mineral-Rich Diet

This diet is designed to support hormone production, reduce estrogenic foods, and provide the nutrients needed for male vitality.

Best Foods to Include

1. **Eggs and grass-fed beef** – Provide cholesterol, a precursor for testosterone
2. **Pumpkin seeds and oysters** – Zinc-rich foods for hormone production
3. **Cruciferous vegetables (broccoli, cauliflower)** – Help detox excess estrogen
4. **Avocados and olive oil** – Healthy fats for hormone synthesis
5. **Dark leafy greens (spinach, kale)** – Magnesium for testosterone and energy
6. **Pomegranate and citrus** – Improve blood flow and antioxidant support
7. **Nuts (brazil nuts, walnuts)** – Contain selenium and essential fats
8. **Chia and flaxseeds** – Hormone-balancing plant foods
9. **Bone broth and collagen** – Support recovery, joint and tissue health
10. **Filtered water and green tea** – Hydration and antioxidant protection

What This Diet Does

> This diet increases the building blocks of testosterone, supports detox of estrogenic compounds, and delivers minerals like zinc, magnesium, and selenium — all crucial for male reproductive health and hormonal balance.

Scientific References for Diet & Testosterone

1. **Pilz, S., et al. (2011)**. *"Vitamin D improves testosterone levels in deficient men." Horm Metab Res, 43(3), 223–225.*
2. **Prasad, A. S., et al. (1996)**. *"Zinc supplementation increases testosterone." Nutrition, 12(5), 344–348.*
3. **Wilborn, C., et al. (2010)**. *"Fenugreek supports male hormonal balance." Int J Sport Nutr Exerc Metab, 20(6), 457–465.*

Lupus (Systemic Lupus Erythematosus – SLE)

Lupus is a chronic autoimmune disease where the immune system attacks the body's own tissues, causing widespread inflammation that can affect the skin, joints, kidneys, brain, and other organs. Natural remedies focus on calming the immune system, reducing inflammation, and supporting organ health — especially when used alongside medical care.

Herbal & Alternative Remedies for Lupus

1. **Turmeric/Curcumin (*Curcuma longa*)**

   - **What it does**: Reduces systemic inflammation and modulates immune responses.

   - **How to use**: 500–1000 mg/day of standardized extract with black pepper.

   Reference:
   Chainani-Wu, N. (2003). *"Safety and anti-inflammatory activity of curcumin."* Alternative Medicine Review, 8(4), 302–320.

2. **Omega-3 Fatty Acids (Fish Oil or Algae-Based EPA/DHA)**

   - **What it does**: Decreases inflammation and may improve joint pain and fatigue.

   - **How to use**: 1000–3000 mg/day of EPA/DHA.

   Reference:
   Arriens, C., et al. (2015). *"Omega-3s improve lupus disease activity."* Lupus, 24(14), 1436–1446.

3. **Vitamin D3**

   - **What it does**: Regulates immune function; often deficient in people with lupus.

   - **How to use**: 2000–5000 IU/day depending on blood levels.

   Reference:
   Ruiz-Irastorza, G., et al. (2008). *"Vitamin D in systemic lupus erythematosus."* Arthritis Research & Therapy, 10(5), R114.

4. **Ashwagandha (*Withania somnifera*)**

   - **What it does**: Adaptogen that helps manage stress, which can trigger flares.

   - **How to use**: 500–1000 mg/day standardized extract.

Reference:
Chandrasekhar, K., et al. (2012). *"Ashwagandha reduces stress and inflammation."* Indian Journal of Psychological Medicine, 34(3), 255–262.

5. Green Tea Extract (EGCG)

- **What it does**: Anti-inflammatory and antioxidant; may help protect organs affected by lupus.

- **How to use**: 250–500 mg/day standardized to EGCG.

Reference:
Ahmed, S., et al. (2005). *"Green tea and its polyphenols in autoimmune diseases."* Journal of Immunology, 175(11), 7615–7622.

6. Probiotics

- **What it does**: Modulates immune response via gut-liver-immune axis.

- **How to use**: 10–20 billion CFUs/day of multi-strain probiotic.

Reference:
Hevia, A., et al. (2014). *"Gut dysbiosis in lupus and role of probiotics."* Journal of Autoimmunity, 52, 1–7.

7. Boswellia (*Boswellia serrata*)

- **What it does**: Natural anti-inflammatory for joint pain and systemic inflammation.

- **How to use**: 300–500 mg 2x/day (standardized to 65% boswellic acids).

Reference:
Sengupta, K., et al. (2008). *"Boswellia in chronic inflammatory conditions."* International Journal of Clinical Pharmacology Research, 28(3), 113–118.

Diet for Lupus Support

Recommended Diet Type: Autoimmune-Calming, Anti-Inflammatory, Organ-Protective Diet

This diet reduces inflammation, supports gut health (linked to immune function), and nourishes vital organs like the kidneys, skin, and joints — which can be affected by lupus.

Best Foods to Include

1. **Fatty fish (salmon, sardines)** – Omega-3s reduce systemic inflammation
2. **Leafy greens and cruciferous vegetables** – Provide antioxidants and folate
3. **Berries and cherries** – Rich in flavonoids that protect blood vessels and joints
4. **Pumpkin seeds and sunflower seeds** – High in zinc and selenium
5. **Turmeric and ginger** – Natural anti-inflammatories
6. **Avocados and olive oil** – Provide healthy fats and support tissue repair
7. **Bone broth and lentils** – Gentle proteins for tissue and immune support
8. **Green tea** – Calms immune system and protects organs
9. **Fermented foods (yogurt, kefir, sauerkraut)** – Improve gut balance and immunity
10. **Filtered water and herbal teas (nettle, chamomile)** – Hydrate and calm inflammation

Why This Diet Works

- Reduces **flare-triggering inflammation**
- Supports **organ protection and healing**, especially kidneys and skin
- Replenishes **immune-regulating nutrients** like vitamin D, zinc, and omega-3s
- Encourages **gut health**, essential for balanced immune response

Scientific References for Diet & Lupus

1. **Arriens, C., et al. (2015)**. *"Omega-3s reduce lupus symptoms." Lupus, 24(14), 1436–1446.*
2. **Ahmed, S., et al. (2005)**. *"Green tea polyphenols in autoimmune disorders." Journal of Immunology, 175(11), 7615–7622.*

3. **Ruiz-Irastorza, G., et al. (2008).** "Vitamin D deficiency linked to lupus flares." Arthritis Research & Therapy, 10(5), R114

Memory Loss (Brain Fog, Forgetfulness, Cognitive Decline)

Memory loss can stem from stress, aging, nutritional deficiencies, poor sleep, or neurological conditions. It may show up as forgetfulness, difficulty concentrating, or mental fog. Natural remedies aim to enhance brain circulation, reduce inflammation, and support neurotransmitter and brain cell health.

Herbal & Alternative Remedies for Memory Loss

1. **Ginkgo Biloba**

   - **What it does**: Enhances circulation to the brain and improves short-term memory and focus.

   - **How to use**: 120–240 mg/day of standardized extract (24% flavone glycosides).

   Reference:
   Weinmann, S., et al. (2010). *"Ginkgo biloba for cognitive impairment and dementia."* Cochrane Database of Systematic Reviews, (2), CD003120.

2. **Bacopa Monnieri (Brahmi)**

   - **What it does**: Improves memory recall, reduces anxiety, and supports learning speed.

   - **How to use**: 300–500 mg/day standardized to bacosides.

   Reference:
   Stough, C., et al. (2001). *"Bacopa improves memory in healthy adults."* Psychopharmacology, 156(4), 481–484.

3. **Lion's Mane Mushroom (*Hericium erinaceus*)**

   - **What it does**: Stimulates nerve growth factor (NGF), helping brain regeneration.

   - **How to use**: 500–1000 mg/day extract or capsules.

   Reference:
   Mori, K., et al. (2009). *"Lion's mane improves mild cognitive impairment."* Phytotherapy Research, 23(3), 367–372.

4. **Rhodiola Rosea**

- **What it does**: Adaptogen that boosts focus, reduces brain fog, and combats fatigue.

- **How to use**: 200–400 mg/day (standardized to rosavins).

Reference:
Darbinyan, V., et al. (2000). *"Rhodiola enhances cognitive performance."* Phytomedicine, 7(5), 365–371.

5. **Omega-3 Fatty Acids (Fish Oil or Algae)**

- **What it does**: Essential for brain structure and function; supports memory and mood.

- **How to use**: 1000–2000 mg/day of combined EPA/DHA.

Reference:
Yurko-Mauro, K., et al. (2010). *"Omega-3s improve cognitive function in aging adults."* Alzheimer's & Dementia, 6(6), 456–464.

6. **Acetyl-L-Carnitine (ALCAR)**

- **What it does**: Boosts brain energy and neurotransmitter activity.

- **How to use**: 500–1500 mg/day in divided doses.

Reference:
Montgomery, S. A., et al. (2003). *"ALCAR in age-related cognitive decline."* International Journal of Clinical Pharmacology Research, 23(2-3), 61–67.

7. **Vitamin B12 (Methylcobalamin)**

- **What it does**: Prevents memory issues caused by deficiency; supports myelin and neurotransmitters.

- **How to use**: 500–1000 mcg/day sublingual or injection under supervision.

Reference:
Moore, E., et al. (2012). *"B12 levels linked to memory loss."* The Journals of Gerontology: Series A, 67(10), 1190–1196.

Diet for Memory Support

Recommended Diet Type: Brain-Boosting, Anti-Inflammatory, Neuroprotective Diet (e.g. MIND Diet)

This diet supports optimal brain health by reducing inflammation, improving blood flow, and fueling cognitive function.

Best Foods to Include

1. **Fatty fish (salmon, mackerel)** – Omega-3s for brain structure and neurotransmission
2. **Blueberries and dark berries** – Rich in flavonoids and antioxidants
3. **Leafy greens (spinach, kale)** – Packed with folate and brain-protective nutrients
4. **Nuts and seeds (especially walnuts)** – Provide vitamin E and brain-supportive fats
5. **Eggs** – High in choline, needed for memory-related neurotransmitters
6. **Avocados and olive oil** – Promote healthy circulation and reduce brain inflammation
7. **Green tea** – Contains L-theanine and EGCG for focus and calm
8. **Pumpkin seeds** – High in magnesium, zinc, and antioxidants
9. **Dark chocolate (70%+ cocoa)** – Enhances cognitive performance via flavonoids
10. **Whole grains and legumes** – Slow-digesting energy for mental stamina

Why This Diet Works

- Enhances **brain plasticity** and slows cognitive decline
- Provides **antioxidants and anti-inflammatories** that protect brain cells
- Fuels **neurotransmitter function** with essential fats, B vitamins, and minerals
- Improves **blood flow** and supports memory formation

Scientific References for Diet & Memory Support

1. **Weinmann, S., et al. (2010)**. *"Ginkgo improves memory and cognition." Cochrane Database, (2), CD003120.*
2. **Mori, K., et al. (2009)**. *"Lion's mane enhances cognitive function." Phytotherapy Research, 23(3), 367–372.*
3. **Yurko-Mauro, K., et al. (2010)**. "Omega-3 fatty acids support brain performance." Alzheimer's & Dementia, 6(6), 456–464.

Menopause Symptoms

Menopause is a natural biological transition marked by the decline of estrogen and progesterone, often accompanied by hot flashes, night sweats, mood swings, sleep disturbances, vaginal dryness, and weight changes. Natural remedies can help balance hormones, ease symptoms, and support overall well-being during this phase.

Herbal & Alternative Remedies for Menopause

1. **Black Cohosh (*Actaea racemosa*)**

    - **What it does**: Relieves hot flashes, mood swings, and sleep disturbances by modulating estrogen receptors.

    - **How to use**: 40–80 mg extract/day.

    Reference:
    Osmers, R., et al. (2005). *"Black cohosh and climacteric complaints: a meta-analysis."* International Journal of Clinical Pharmacology and Therapeutics, 43(3), 134–138.

2. **Red Clover (*Trifolium pratense*)**

    - **What it does**: Contains plant-based estrogens (isoflavones) that ease hot flashes and vaginal dryness.

    - **How to use**: 40–80 mg/day of standardized isoflavones.

    Reference:
    Lethaby, A., et al. (2007). *"Phytoestrogens for vasomotor menopausal symptoms."* Cochrane Database of Systematic Reviews, (4), CD001395.

3. **Maca Root (*Lepidium meyenii*)**

    - **What it does**: Supports hormone balance, libido, and mood without containing estrogen.

    - **How to use**: 1500–3000 mg/day of gelatinized root powder.

    Reference:
    Brooks, N. A., et al. (2008). *"Maca reduces blood pressure and depression in postmenopausal women."* Menopause, 15(4), 707–712.

4. **Evening Primrose Oil (*Oenothera biennis*)**

    - **What it does**: May reduce hot flashes and improve skin hydration.

    - **How to use**: 500–1000 mg capsule, 2x/day.

Reference:

Farzaneh, F., et al. (2013). *"A randomized controlled trial of evening primrose oil in menopausal hot flashes."* Archives of Gynecology and Obstetrics, 288(5), 1075–1079.

5. **Dong Quai (*Angelica sinensis*)**

   - **What it does**: Traditional Chinese herb for hormonal balance and circulation.

   - **How to use**: 1000–1500 mg/day or as part of a blended formula.

   Reference:

   Wuttke, W., et al. (2003). *"Phytoestrogens for hormone replacement therapy?"* Journal of Steroid Biochemistry and Molecular Biology, 83(1–5), 133–147.

6. **Ashwagandha (*Withania somnifera*)**

   - **What it does**: Reduces stress, anxiety, and supports thyroid and adrenal hormones.

   - **How to use**: 500–1000 mg/day standardized extract.

   Reference:

   Chandrasekhar, K., et al. (2012). *"Stress-relieving and hormone-supportive effects of ashwagandha."* Indian Journal of Psychological Medicine, 34(3), 255–262.

7. **Flaxseed (*Linum usitatissimum*)**

   - **What it does**: Contains lignans (phytoestrogens) that may reduce hot flashes and improve mood.

   - **How to use**: 1–2 tbsp ground daily in smoothies, yogurt, or oats.

   - **Reference:**
     Pruthi, S., et al. (2007). *"Pilot study of flaxseed for the treatment of hot flashes."* Journal of the Society for Integrative Oncology, 5(3), 106–112.

Diet for Menopause Symptom Relief

Recommended Diet Type: Hormone-Balancing, Phytoestrogen-Rich Mediterranean Diet This diet emphasizes plant-based estrogens, healthy fats, and anti-inflammatory foods to balance hormones, reduce hot flashes, and support mood, metabolism, and bone health.

Best Foods to Include

1. **Flaxseeds and sesame seeds** – Rich in lignans (natural estrogen-like compounds)
2. **Soy products (tofu, tempeh)** – Contain isoflavones to ease hormonal symptoms
3. **Leafy greens** – High in calcium and magnesium for bone and mood support
4. **Berries** – Packed with antioxidants to reduce oxidative stress and hot flashes
5. **Fatty fish** – Omega-3s help with mood, inflammation, and heart health
6. **Whole grains (quinoa, oats)** – Balance blood sugar and provide B vitamins
7. **Nuts (especially almonds and walnuts)** – Healthy fats and vitamin E
8. **Avocados and olive oil** – Support hormone production and skin health
9. **Chickpeas and lentils** – Fiber-rich and a good source of phytoestrogens
10. **Herbal teas (red clover, chamomile)** – Naturally calming and hormone-supportive

Why This Diet Works

- Boosts **plant-based estrogens** to ease hormonal shifts

- Supports **neurotransmitters and mood** with B vitamins and magnesium

- Balances blood sugar to prevent **energy crashes and irritability**

- Supports **heart, bone, and brain health** — all vulnerable post-menopause

Scientific References for Diet & Menopause

1. **Messina, M. J. (2014)**. *"Soy foods, isoflavones, and the health of postmenopausal women." American Journal of Clinical Nutrition, 100(Suppl_1), 423S–430S.*
   ➤ Found that soy isoflavones significantly reduce hot flashes and improve bone density.

2. **Pan, Y., et al. (2009)**. *"Dietary fiber and risk of breast cancer in postmenopausal women." American Journal of Clinical Nutrition, 90(3), 688–697.*
   ➤ Fiber-rich, plant-based diets modulate estrogen levels and reduce menopause-related risk factors.

3. **Sacks, F. M., et al. (2001)**. "DASH and Mediterranean-style diets for cardiovascular risk in postmenopausal women." New England Journal of Medicine, 344(1), 3–10.
   ➤ These diets lower blood pressure and inflammation, supporting overall menopausal health.

Menstrual Cramps (Dysmenorrhea)

Menstrual cramps are caused by contractions of the uterus triggered by prostaglandins — hormone-like substances that cause pain and inflammation. While over-the-counter painkillers are common, many women find lasting relief using natural remedies that reduce inflammation and support hormonal balance.

Herbal & Alternative Remedies for Menstrual Cramps

1. **Cramp Bark (*Viburnum opulus*)**

   o **What it does**: A traditional uterine relaxant that soothes spasms and reduces cramping.

   o **How to use**: 1–2 mL tincture every 3–4 hours as needed or 500–1000 mg capsule twice daily.

   Reference:
   Mills, S., & Bone, K. (2000). *Principles and Practice of Phytotherapy: Modern Herbal Medicine.* Churchill Livingstone.

2. **Ginger (*Zingiber officinale*)**

   o **What it does**: Anti-inflammatory and pain-relieving; reduces prostaglandin production.

   o **How to use**: 750–2000 mg/day of ginger extract or 2–3 cups of ginger tea per day during menstruation.

   Reference:
   Rahnama, P., et al. (2012). *"Effect of Zingiber officinale R. rhizomes (ginger) on pain relief in primary dysmenorrhea."* BMC Complementary and Alternative Medicine, 12, 92.

3. **Cinnamon (*Cinnamomum verum*)**

   o **What it does**: Anti-inflammatory and antispasmodic properties that relieve menstrual pain and bleeding.

   o **How to use**: 1000–1500 mg cinnamon powder daily or 1–2 cups cinnamon tea.

   Reference:
   Jaafarpour, M., et al. (2015). *"The effect of cinnamon on primary dysmenorrhea: a randomized, double-blind clinical trial."* Iranian Red Crescent Medical Journal, 17(4), e27032.

4. **Vitex (*Vitex agnus-castus*)**

   - **What it does**: Balances hormones by supporting progesterone production and reducing estrogen dominance.

   - **How to use**: 400–1000 mg/day standardized extract; take consistently for at least 3 months.

   Reference:
   van Die, M. D., et al. (2013). *"Vitex agnus-castus extracts for female reproductive disorders: a systematic review of clinical trials."* Planta Medica, 79(07), 562–575.

5. **Evening Primrose Oil (*Oenothera biennis*)**

   - **What it does**: Rich in GLA, helps reduce uterine inflammation and hormonal imbalances.

   - **How to use**: 500–1000 mg capsule once or twice daily.

   Reference:
   Kazemian, A., et al. (2013). *"Effect of evening primrose oil on the severity of cyclical mastalgia."* Archives of Gynecology and Obstetrics, 288(4), 845–850.

6. **Magnesium (citrate or glycinate)**

   - **What it does**: Relaxes smooth muscle tissue and helps regulate prostaglandin production.

   - **How to use**: 200–400 mg/day; begin 1–2 days before menstruation and continue through the cycle.

   Reference:
   Walker, A. F., et al. (2001). *"Magnesium supplementation alleviates premenstrual symptoms of fluid retention."* Journal of Women's Health & Gender-Based Medicine, 10(4), 373–378.

Diet for Menstrual Cramp Relief

Recommended Diet Type: Hormone-Balancing Anti-Inflammatory Diet

This diet focuses on reducing prostaglandin activity, supporting liver detoxification of excess estrogen, and increasing intake of anti-inflammatory nutrients and magnesium-rich foods.

Best Foods to Include

1. **Leafy greens** (spinach, kale) – Provide calcium and magnesium for muscle relaxation

2. **Flaxseeds** – Rich in lignans that help balance estrogen levels

3. **Fatty fish** (salmon, sardines) – Omega-3s help lower prostaglandin production

4. **Avocados** – Provide potassium and healthy fats for hormonal support

5. **Berries** – Contain antioxidants that reduce inflammation

6. **Nuts and seeds** (pumpkin, sunflower, chia) – Rich in zinc and magnesium

7. **Turmeric** – Anti-inflammatory spice that reduces uterine inflammation

8. **Beans and legumes** – High in fiber to help eliminate excess estrogen

9. **Quinoa and brown rice** – Complex carbs that stabilize blood sugar and mood

10. **Dark chocolate (70%+)** – Contains magnesium and improves mood

Why This Diet Works

11. Reduces **inflammation and prostaglandin production**, the root cause of cramps

12. Supports **hormonal detoxification** through liver-friendly foods

13. Provides **key minerals** like magnesium and calcium for uterine relaxation

14. Helps **balance estrogen dominance**, which can worsen symptoms

Scientific References for Diet & Menstrual Cramps

1. Nillni, Y. I., et al. (2009). *"The role of nutrition in the etiology and management of dysmenorrhea."* Clinical Obstetrics and Gynecology, 52(3), 610–620.

2. Deutch, B. (1995). *"Menstrual pain in Danish women correlated with low n-3 polyunsaturated fatty acid intake."* European Journal of Clinical Nutrition, 49(7), 508–516.

3. Obeidat, B. A., et al. (2012). *"Premenstrual symptoms and vitamin D levels in healthy women."* Archives of Gynecology and Obstetrics, 285(6), 1535–1539.

Motion Sickness

Motion sickness is a condition where movement — especially in vehicles, boats, or planes — triggers nausea, dizziness, cold sweats, and vomiting. It's caused by conflicting signals between the inner ear, eyes, and brain. Natural remedies aim to calm the nervous system, stabilize balance, and reduce nausea.

Herbal & Alternative Remedies for Motion Sickness

1. **Ginger Root (*Zingiber officinale*) – Tea, Capsule, or Candy**

   - **What it does**: Calms the stomach, reduces nausea, and improves vestibular stability.

   - **How to use**: 500–1000 mg capsule 30 minutes before travel, or 1–2 cups tea.

   Reference:
   Grøntved, A., & Hentzer, E. (1986). *"Ginger's effectiveness against motion-induced nausea."* Acta Otolaryngologica, 102(1-2), 124–129.

2. **Peppermint (*Mentha piperita*) – Tea or Aromatherapy**

   - **What it does**: Relieves nausea and settles the digestive system.

   - **How to use**: Inhale peppermint essential oil or drink 1–2 cups peppermint tea.

   Reference:
   Pittler, M. H., & Ernst, E. (1998). *"Peppermint oil in GI discomfort and nausea."* Phytomedicine, 5(4), 231–235.

3. **Acupressure (P6 / Nei-Kuan Point on Wrist)**

   - **What it does**: Stimulates a pressure point that reduces nausea and vomiting.

   - **How to use**: Apply pressure 2–3 finger-widths below the wrist crease for 1–2 minutes; use acupressure wristbands as needed.

   Reference:
   Dundee, J. W., et al. (1988). *"P6 acupressure reduces motion-induced nausea."* Anaesthesia, 43(6), 456–458.

4. **Vitamin B6 (Pyridoxine)**

- **What it does**: Helps reduce nausea and supports the nervous system.

- **How to use**: 25–50 mg up to 3x/day, especially before and during travel.

Reference:
Sahakian, V., et al. (1991). *"Vitamin B6 in nausea treatment."* Obstetrics & Gynecology, 78(1), 33–36.

5. **Chamomile (*Matricaria recutita*) – Tea or Tincture**

- **What it does**: Soothes the stomach and calms anxiety-related nausea.

- **How to use**: Drink 1–2 cups tea before travel or use ½–1 dropperful tincture in water.

Reference:
McKay, D. L., & Blumberg, J. B. (2006). *"Chamomile's soothing GI properties."* Phytotherapy Research, 20(7), 519–530.

6. **Lemon Balm (*Melissa officinalis*) – Tea or Extract**

- **What it does**: Mild calming herb that reduces anxiety and nausea.

- **How to use**: 1–2 cups/day or 300–600 mg extract before travel.

Reference:
Kennedy, D. O., et al. (2003). *"Lemon balm improves mood and calms nerves."* Psychosomatic Medicine, 65(4), 607–613.

7. **CBD Oil (Cannabidiol)**

- **What it does**: Reduces nausea and anxiety, which can trigger motion sickness.

- **How to use**: 5–15 mg sublingually 30 minutes before travel.

Reference:
Rock, E. M., et al. (2011). *"Cannabinoids for nausea and vomiting."* British Journal of Pharmacology, 163(7), 1411–1422.

Diet for Motion Sickness Support

Recommended Diet Type: Digestive-Calming, Low-Glycemic, Anti-Nausea Diet

This diet helps calm the stomach, regulate blood sugar, and avoid triggers that exacerbate motion-induced nausea and dizziness.

Best Foods to Include

1. **Plain crackers or toast** – Settles the stomach and prevents hunger-triggered nausea
2. **Bananas and applesauce** – Gentle, non-acidic fruits with easy digestion
3. **Ginger tea or chews** – Anti-nausea and warming
4. **Oats and rice** – Bland, steady-carb foods that stabilize digestion
5. **Chamomile and peppermint teas** – Reduce queasiness and relax the GI tract
6. **Yogurt (unsweetened)** – Balances the gut and soothes digestion
7. **Almonds or pumpkin seeds** – Protein and minerals without heaviness
8. **Cucumber and celery** – Hydrating and mild
9. **Herbal infusions (lemon balm, fennel)** – Calm nerves and reduce stomach spasms
10. **Water with lemon (small amount)** – Keeps you hydrated without fullness

Why This Diet Works

- Avoids **heavy, greasy, or acidic foods** that trigger nausea
- Provides **easily digestible, calming foods** that keep the stomach settled
- Includes **herbs and teas** that soothe the gut and calm the nervous system
- Helps maintain **steady blood sugar**, preventing dizziness and nausea

Scientific References for Diet & Motion Sickness

1. **Grøntved, A., & Hentzer, E. (1986)**. *"Ginger in motion sickness." Acta Otolaryngol, 102(1-2), 124–129.*
2. **Dundee, J. W., et al. (1988)**. *"P6 acupressure in motion-induced nausea." Anaesthesia, 43(6), 456–458.*
3. **Sahakian, V., et al. (1991)**. *"Vitamin B6 reduces nausea severity." Obstetrics & Gynecology, 78(1), 33–36.*

Mood Swings

Mood swings refer to sudden, often unpredictable changes in emotional state — from irritability or sadness to calm or happiness. They can be caused by hormonal changes (PMS, menopause), blood sugar imbalances, stress, or mental health conditions. Natural remedies aim to support hormonal balance, stabilize neurotransmitters, and reduce stress.

Herbal & Alternative Remedies for Mood Swings

1. **Maca Root (*Lepidium meyenii*)**

   - **What it does**: Balances hormones, especially during PMS, menopause, and stress.

   - **How to use**: 1.5–3 grams/day in powder or capsule form.

   Reference:
   Brooks, N. A., et al. (2008). *"Maca improves mood and hormone balance."* Menopause, 15(6), 1157–1162.

2. **St. John's Wort (*Hypericum perforatum*)**

   - **What it does**: Natural antidepressant that supports serotonin balance.

   - **How to use**: 300 mg extract (standardized to 0.3% hypericin) 2–3x/day.

   Reference:
   Linde, K., et al. (2005). *"St. John's Wort for depression."* Cochrane Database of Systematic Reviews, (2), CD000448.

3. **Ashwagandha (*Withania somnifera*)**

   - **What it does**: Adaptogen that lowers cortisol and reduces emotional instability.

   - **How to use**: 300–600 mg/day of standardized extract.

   Reference:
   Chandrasekhar, K., et al. (2012). *"Ashwagandha reduces stress and improves mood."* Indian Journal of Psychological Medicine, 34(3), 255–262.

4. **Vitex (Chaste Tree Berry – *Vitex agnus-castus*)**

   - **What it does**: Supports progesterone production and balances menstrual cycle mood shifts.

   - **How to use**: 20–40 mg/day standardized extract.

Reference:
Loch, E. G., et al. (2000). *"Vitex reduces PMS symptoms and mood swings."* British Journal of Phytotherapy, 5(2), 29–33.

5. Rhodiola Rosea

- **What it does**: Adaptogen that boosts resilience to emotional and physical stress.

- **How to use**: 200–400 mg/day (standardized to rosavins and salidrosides).

Reference:
Darbinyan, V., et al. (2000). *"Rhodiola improves mood and cognitive function."* Phytomedicine, 7(5), 365–371.

6. Magnesium (Citrate or Glycinate)

- **What it does**: Calms the nervous system, supports mood stability, and reduces irritability.

- **How to use**: 300–400 mg/day.

Reference:
Eby, G. A., & Eby, K. L. (2006). *"Magnesium for mood stabilization."* Medical Hypotheses, 67(2), 362–370.

7. L-Theanine (Green Tea Amino Acid)

- **What it does**: Promotes relaxation without sedation and improves focus.

- **How to use**: 100–200 mg/day or 1–2 cups green tea.

Reference:
Lu, K., et al. (2004). *"L-theanine and mood regulation."* Biological Psychology, 77(2), 113–122.

Diet for Mood Stability Support

Recommended Diet Type: Mood-Stabilizing, Hormone-Balancing, Blood Sugar-Supportive Diet

This diet reduces blood sugar crashes, supports healthy neurotransmitter production, and helps regulate hormones linked to mood.

Best Foods to Include

1. **Leafy greens and broccoli** – Rich in B vitamins and magnesium
2. **Salmon and sardines** – Omega-3s for mood and brain support
3. **Pumpkin seeds and almonds** – Provide zinc and healthy fats
4. **Bananas and avocados** – Contain mood-stabilizing B6 and tryptophan
5. **Fermented foods (yogurt, kimchi, sauerkraut)** – Support gut-brain balance
6. **Whole grains (oats, brown rice, quinoa)** – Slow-burning carbs that stabilize blood sugar
7. **Eggs and lean proteins** – Provide amino acids to build serotonin and dopamine
8. **Berries and citrus fruits** – High in vitamin C and antioxidants
9. **Green tea and herbal teas (chamomile, holy basil)** – Promote calm without sedating
10. **Filtered water** – Keeps mood-stabilizing minerals circulating

Why This Diet Works

- Supports **neurotransmitter production** (serotonin, dopamine)
- Balances **blood sugar levels**, preventing mood crashes
- Reduces **inflammation and oxidative stress** affecting the brain
- Enhances **gut health**, which plays a key role in emotional regulation

Scientific References for Diet & Mood Swings

1. **Brooks, N. A., et al. (2008).** *"Maca reduces mood variability." Menopause, 15(6), 1157–1162.*
2. **Linde, K., et al. (2005).** *"St. John's Wort improves depressive symptoms." Cochrane Database, (2), CD000448.*
3. **Eby, G. A., & Eby, K. L. (2006).** "Magnesium stabilizes mood." Medical Hypotheses, 67(2), 362–370.

Non-Alcoholic Fatty Liver Disease (NAFLD)

NAFLD is a condition where excess fat builds up in the liver without alcohol being the cause. It's often linked to insulin resistance, obesity, high triglycerides, or poor diet. Natural remedies aim to reduce liver fat, support detox, and improve metabolic health.

Herbal & Alternative Remedies for NAFLD

1. **Milk Thistle (*Silybum marianum*) – Capsule or Tea**

    o **What it does**: Supports liver regeneration, reduces inflammation, and helps detoxify fat accumulation.

    o **How to use**: 150–300 mg/day (standardized to 70–80% silymarin).

    Reference:
    Federico, A., et al. (2014). *"Milk thistle improves liver markers in NAFLD."* World Journal of Gastroenterology, 20(36), 12811–12819.

2. **Turmeric (Curcumin)**

    o **What it does**: Anti-inflammatory and antioxidant; reduces liver fat and inflammation.

    o **How to use**: 500–1000 mg/day with black pepper or healthy fats for absorption.

    Reference:
    Panahi, Y., et al. (2017). *"Curcumin significantly improves liver enzymes in NAFLD."* Phytotherapy Research, 31(11), 1829–1835

3. **Dandelion Root – Tea or Tincture**

    o **What it does**: Promotes bile flow and supports liver detoxification.

    o **How to use**: 1–2 cups/day tea or 500 mg extract/day.

    Reference:
    Clare, B. A., et al. (2009). *"Dandelion aids hepatic function and detoxification."* J Altern Complement Med, 15(8), 817–828.

4. **Artichoke Leaf (*Cynara scolymus*) – Extract**

    o **What it does**: Enhances bile production, lowers cholesterol, and improves liver health.

    o **How to use**: 300–640 mg/day standardized extract.

    Reference:
    Luper, S. (1999). *"Artichoke shows hepatoprotective effects."* Alternative Medicine Review, 4(6), 372–386.

5. Berberine – Capsule

- o **What it does**: Improves insulin sensitivity and reduces fat in the liver.

- o **How to use**: 500 mg 2–3x/day.

Reference:
Zhang, Y., et al. (2008). *"Berberine reduces hepatic fat in NAFLD."* Metabolism, 57(5), 712–717.

6. Green Tea Extract (EGCG)

- o **What it does**: Reduces oxidative stress and liver fat accumulation.

- o **How to use**: 400–800 mg/day or drink 2–3 cups brewed green tea.

Reference:
Sakata, R., et al. (2013). *"Green tea improves fat metabolism and liver markers."* Journal of Nutritional Biochemistry, 24(6), 943–950.

7. Alpha-Lipoic Acid (ALA)

- o **What it does**: Powerful antioxidant that helps reverse fatty liver changes.

- o **How to use**: 300–600 mg/day.

Reference:
Zhang, Q., et al. (2012). *"ALA improves liver enzymes in metabolic conditions."* Free Radical Biology and Medicine, 53(2), 361–373.

Diet for NAFLD Reversal

Recommended Diet Type: Mediterranean, Anti-Inflammatory, Liver-Supportive Diet

This diet emphasizes healthy fats, fiber, antioxidants, and foods that stabilize blood sugar to reduce liver fat accumulation.

Best Foods to Include

1. **Fatty fish (salmon, sardines)** – Omega-3s reduce liver fat
2. **Leafy greens and cruciferous vegetables** – Support detox and reduce inflammation
3. **Avocados and olives** – Healthy monounsaturated fats
4. **Nuts and seeds (especially walnuts and flaxseeds)** – Help reduce triglycerides
5. **Berries and citrus fruits** – Rich in antioxidants
6. **Legumes and lentils** – Provide fiber and regulate blood sugar
7. **Whole grains (quinoa, oats, brown rice)** – Low-glycemic carbs
8. **Green tea and turmeric** – Fight inflammation and fat buildup
9. **Beets and carrots** – Contain liver-supporting compounds
10. **Filtered water and lemon water** – Aid liver filtration and digestion

Why This Diet Works

- Reduces **fat buildup in the liver**
- Balances **insulin and blood sugar levels**, key in NAFLD
- Increases **antioxidant protection and detoxification**
- Supports **gut health**, which influences liver inflammation

Scientific References for Diet & Fatty Liver Disease

1. **Panahi, Y., et al. (2017)**. *"Curcumin improves NAFLD indicators."* Phytother Res, 31(11), 1829–1835.
2. **Federico, A., et al. (2014)**. *"Milk thistle improves liver function in NAFLD patients."* World J Gastroenterol, 20(36), 12811–12819.
3. **Zhang, Y., et al. (2008)**. *"Berberine reduces liver fat and metabolic dysfunction."* Metabolism, 57(5), 712–717.

PCOS (Polycystic Ovary Syndrome)

PCOS is a hormonal disorder affecting women, characterized by irregular periods, ovarian cysts, acne, weight gain, and insulin resistance. It often includes elevated androgens and can lead to fertility issues. Natural remedies aim to balance hormones, regulate cycles, improve insulin sensitivity, and support metabolism.

Herbal & Alternative Remedies for PCOS

1. **Inositol (Myo- & D-Chiro-Inositol)**

   - **What it does**: Improves insulin sensitivity, supports ovulation, and reduces androgen levels.

   - **How to use**: 2000–4000 mg/day (usually in a 40:1 Myo:D-Chiro ratio).

   Reference:
   Genazzani, A. D., et al. (2018). *"Inositols in PCOS treatment."* Gynecological Endocrinology, 34(7), 545–550.

2. **Spearmint Tea**

   - **What it does**: Reduces testosterone levels, improves hirsutism and acne.

   - **How to use**: 1–2 cups/day, steeped 5–10 minutes.

   Reference:
   Grant, P. (2010). *"Spearmint herbal tea has significant anti-androgen effects in PCOS."* Phytotherapy Research, 24(2), 186–188.

3. **Vitex / Chaste Tree (*Vitex agnus-castus*)**

   - **What it does**: Balances the pituitary gland, supports ovulation, regulates cycles.

   - **How to use**: 400–1000 mg/day or 1 dropperful tincture in the morning.

   Reference:
   Jelodar, G., et al. (2018). *"Effect of Vitex agnus-castus on PCOS in rats."* Avicenna Journal of Phytomedicine, 8(6), 567–576.

4. **Berberine**

   - **What it does**: Improves insulin resistance and lowers androgen levels; similar effects to metformin.

- **How to use**: 500 mg, 2–3x/day before meals.

Reference:
Wei, W., et al. (2012). *"Berberine improves insulin resistance in PCOS women."* Clinical Endocrinology, 77(6), 823–830.

5. Maca Root (*Lepidium meyenii*)

- **What it does**: Supports hormone balance, energy, and mood without mimicking estrogen.

- **How to use**: 1500–3000 mg/day of gelatinized maca powder or capsules.

Reference:
Brooks, N. A., et al. (2008). *"Maca's effect on mood and hormonal balance in menopausal women."* Menopause, 15(4), 707–712.

6. Cinnamon (*Cinnamomum cassia*)

- **What it does**: Helps reduce insulin resistance and regulate menstrual cycles.

- **How to use**: 1000–1500 mg/day of extract or ½–1 tsp powder in food.

Reference:
Wang, J., et al. (2007). *"Cinnamon extract improves menstrual cyclicity in PCOS."* Fertility and Sterility, 88(6), 1749–1754.

7. Omega-3 Fatty Acids (Fish Oil or Algae Oil)

- **What it does**: Lowers inflammation and testosterone, supports insulin sensitivity.

- **How to use**: 1000–2000 mg/day of EPA/DHA.

Reference:
Khani, B., et al. (2017). *"Fish oil supplementation improves PCOS metabolic parameters."* Caspian Journal of Internal Medicine, 8(4), 261–267.

Diet for PCOS Relief

Recommended Diet Type: Low-Glycemic, Anti-Androgenic, Hormone-Balancing Diet

This diet improves insulin sensitivity, supports hormone production, and reduces inflammation. It avoids refined carbs, sugar, dairy (if sensitive), and processed foods that can trigger androgen dominance.

Best Foods to Include

1. **Leafy greens and cruciferous vegetables** – Support estrogen detox and hormone balance
2. **Berries and citrus fruits** – Antioxidants and fiber support insulin sensitivity
3. **Legumes and lentils** – Rich in fiber and slow-digesting carbs
4. **Pumpkin and flax seeds** – Provide healthy fats and hormone-regulating lignans
5. **Wild-caught salmon and sardines** – Omega-3s reduce inflammation and support hormone health
6. **Avocados and olive oil** – Promote healthy fats and stabilize blood sugar
7. **Quinoa and oats** – Low glycemic, fiber-rich complex carbs
8. **Spearmint tea and green tea** – Naturally lower androgens and inflammation
9. **Fermented foods** – Improve gut balance, which supports hormone regulation
10. **Filtered water and herbal teas** – Help flush out excess hormones and support hydration

Why This Diet Works

- Reduces **insulin resistance**, a core driver of PCOS
- Lowers **androgen production** by avoiding high-glycemic and inflammatory foods
- Balances **hormones naturally** through fiber, phytonutrients, and good fats

- Promotes **regular ovulation and stable cycles**

Scientific References for Diet & PCOS

1. **Douglas, C. C., et al. (2006).** *"Nutritional strategies for insulin resistance in PCOS." Journal of the American Dietetic Association, 106(4), 537–545.*
   ➤ Low-glycemic diets significantly improve insulin sensitivity and menstrual regularity.

2. **Moran, L. J., et al. (2013).** *"Dietary composition in the treatment of PCOS." American Journal of Clinical Nutrition, 97(3), 667–677.*
   ➤ High-protein, low-glycemic diets with healthy fats improve ovulation and reduce androgen levels.

3. **Khani, B., et al. (2017).** *"Omega-3 improves lipid profiles and inflammation in PCOS." Caspian Journal of Internal Medicine, 8(4), 261–267.*
   ➤ Omega-3 supplementation improves metabolic and hormonal markers in PCOS patients.

Plantar Fasciitis

Plantar fasciitis is inflammation of the thick band of tissue (plantar fascia) that runs along the bottom of the foot, causing sharp heel pain — especially first thing in the morning or after long periods of standing. Natural remedies focus on reducing inflammation, promoting tissue healing, and relieving tension in the fascia.

Herbal & Alternative Remedies for Plantar Fasciitis

1. **Turmeric/Curcumin (*Curcuma longa*)**

    - **What it does**: Reduces inflammation in connective tissue and relieves pain.

    - **How to use**: 500–1000 mg/day of standardized extract with black pepper for absorption.

    Reference:
    Belcaro, G., et al. (2010). *"Efficacy of curcumin in pain and inflammation management."* Panminerva Medica, 52(2 Suppl 1), 55–62.

2. **Boswellia (*Boswellia serrata*)**

    - **What it does**: Reduces inflammatory enzymes, easing connective tissue pain.

    - **How to use**: 300–500 mg extract 2x/day (standardized to 65% boswellic acids).

    Reference:
    Sengupta, K., et al. (2008). *"Boswellia extract in joint pain and soft tissue inflammation."* International Journal of Clinical Pharmacology Research, 28(3), 113–118

3. **Epsom Salt (Magnesium Sulfate) Foot Soaks**

    - **What it does**: Relaxes muscles and fascia, eases soreness.

    - **How to use**: ½–1 cup in warm water; soak feet 15–20 min daily.

    Reference:
    Waryasz, G. R., & McDermott, A. Y. (2008). *"Epsom salt and recovery from inflammation."* Journal of Strength and Conditioning Research, 22(3), 869–876.

4. **Capsaicin Cream (Topical)**

    - **What it does**: Temporarily desensitizes pain receptors in the heel.

- **How to use**: Apply 0.025–0.1% capsaicin cream to heel 2–4x/day.

Reference:
Deal, C. L., et al. (1991). *"Capsaicin cream for treatment of pain."* Clinical Therapeutics, 13(3), 383–395.

5. **Arnica (*Arnica montana*) – Topical Cream or Gel**

   - **What it does**: Reduces swelling and bruising in soft tissue.

   - **How to use**: Apply thin layer to affected area 2–3x/day.

   Reference:
   Knuesel, O., et al. (2002). *"Efficacy of topical arnica in soft-tissue injuries."* Advances in Therapy, 19(5), 209–218.

6. **Massage with Essential Oils (Peppermint, Eucalyptus, Lavender)**

   - **What it does**: Improves circulation and eases muscle tightness.

   - **How to use**: Dilute essential oil in a carrier oil and massage arch of foot and heel.

   Reference:
   Lakhan, S. E., et al. (2016). *"Massage therapy for pain relief: a meta-analysis."* Pain Medicine, 17(7), 1241–1247.

7. **Acupressure or Reflexology**

   - **What it does**: Stimulates blood flow and relieves pressure in the feet.

   - **How to use**: Apply firm pressure along heel and arch using fingers or a massage tool.

   Reference:
   Ernst, E., & Posadzki, P. (2011). *"Reflexology for pain management."* Maturitas, 68(2), 116–120.

Diet for Plantar Fasciitis Relief

Recommended Diet Type: Anti-Inflammatory, Tissue-Healing Diet

This diet helps reduce systemic inflammation that contributes to chronic pain and supports collagen and tissue repair in ligaments, tendons, and fascia.

Best Foods to Include

1. **Leafy greens (spinach, kale)** – High in anti-inflammatory compounds and magnesium
2. **Fatty fish (salmon, sardines)** – Omega-3s to reduce pain and inflammation
3. **Berries and cherries** – Packed with antioxidants to fight oxidative stress
4. **Bone broth** – High in collagen and amino acids for tissue regeneration
5. **Turmeric and ginger** – Potent natural anti-inflammatories
6. **Nuts and seeds (especially walnuts, flaxseed)** – Healthy fats and anti-inflammatory benefits
7. **Sweet potatoes and quinoa** – Anti-inflammatory complex carbs
8. **Citrus fruits and bell peppers** – High in vitamin C for collagen synthesis
9. **Pumpkin seeds** – Rich in zinc and magnesium for tissue health
10. **Filtered water and herbal teas** – Keep tissues hydrated and reduce muscle tension

Why This Diet Works

- Reduces **inflammation in connective tissue** and soft tissue
- Provides nutrients like **vitamin C, magnesium, and collagen** to support fascia repair
- Supports **circulation and hydration** for recovery and pain relief
- Helps with **weight management**, which reduces pressure on the plantar fascia

Scientific References for Diet & Plantar Fasciitis

1. **Zhang, Y., et al. (2014).** *"Anti-inflammatory diet and musculoskeletal pain." Nutrition Journal, 13(1), 14.*
   ➤ Diets rich in anti-inflammatory nutrients improve outcomes in chronic pain conditions.
2. **Sengupta, K., et al. (2008).** *"Boswellia and soft tissue recovery." International Journal of Clinical Pharmacology Research, 28(3), 113–*

118.

> Boswellia significantly reduced inflammation in connective tissue.

3. **Knuesel, O., et al. (2002).** *"Topical arnica effective for pain and inflammation." Advances in Therapy, 19(5), 209–218.*

> Arnica gel helped reduce inflammation in localized soft-tissue injuries.

Pneumonia

Pneumonia is an infection that inflames the air sacs in one or both lungs, which may fill with fluid or pus. It can be caused by bacteria, viruses, or fungi. Symptoms include cough, fever, chills, and difficulty breathing. Natural remedies can help support lung function, reduce inflammation, and fight infection — but they should **always be used alongside medical care**, not as a substitute.

Herbal & Alternative Remedies for Pneumonia

1. **Echinacea (*Echinacea purpurea*)**
   - **What it does**: Enhances immune response and helps the body fight infections.
   - **How to use**: 300–500 mg extract 2–3x/day or 1 dropperful tincture 3x/day.

   Reference:
   Barrett, B., et al. (2003). *"Echinacea's effect on respiratory infections."* Annals of Internal Medicine, 137(12), 939–946.

2. **Licorice Root (*Glycyrrhiza glabra*) – Tea or Syrup**
   - **What it does**: Soothes the respiratory tract and acts as an expectorant.
   - **How to use**: 1–2 cups tea/day or 400–800 mg extract 2x/day. Avoid with high blood pressure.

   Reference:
   Wang, Y., et al. (2015). *"Pharmacological properties of licorice in lung infections."* Acta Pharmaceutica Sinica B, 5(4), 310–315.

3. **Oregano Oil (Oral Capsules)**
   - **What it does**: Natural antibacterial and antiviral; may support clearing lung infections.
   - **How to use**: 150–300 mg/day enteric-coated capsules or diluted oil under tongue (consult practitioner).

   Reference:
   Force, M., et al. (2000). *"Oregano oil shows antimicrobial activity."* Phytotherapy Research, 14(3), 213–218.

4. **Thyme (*Thymus vulgaris*) – Tea or Steam**
   - **What it does**: Expectorant and bronchodilator; helps clear mucus and open airways.

- **How to use**: 1–2 cups tea/day or add to steam inhalation.

Reference:
Benedek, B., et al. (2008). *"Thyme extract in bronchial conditions."* Planta Medica, 74(9), 1170–1175.

5. **Mullein (*Verbascum thapsus*) – Tea or Tincture**
   - **What it does**: Soothes inflamed lungs, helps remove mucus.
   - **How to use**: 1–2 cups tea/day or 1–2 mL tincture 2x/day.

Reference:
Thomsen, M. (2013). *"Medicinal Plants for Respiratory Conditions."* HerbalGram, 100, 54–63.

6. **N-Acetylcysteine (NAC)**
   - **What it does**: Breaks down mucus and boosts lung glutathione, aiding detoxification.
   - **How to use**: 600–1200 mg/day.

Reference:
Aldini, G., et al. (2018). *"NAC for lung health and detoxification."* Pharmacological Research, 134, 1–7.

7. **Andrographis (*Andrographis paniculata*)**
   - **What it does**: Antiviral and anti-inflammatory; supports immunity during respiratory infections.
   - **How to use**: 400–800 mg/day standardized to 10–30% andrographolides.

Reference:
Poolsup, N., et al. (2004). *"Andrographis reduces severity of respiratory infections."* Phytomedicine, 11(6), 385–393.

Diet for Pneumonia Support

Recommended Diet Type: Immune-Boosting, Mucus-Clearing, Anti-Inflammatory Diet

This diet supports immune function, helps clear mucus, and reduces inflammation in the lungs.

Best Foods to Include

1. **Garlic and onions** – Natural antimicrobials that support lung and immune function
2. **Bone broth** – Hydrating and rich in amino acids for tissue repair
3. **Leafy greens and cruciferous veggies** – Provide immune-enhancing vitamins A, C, and K
4. **Citrus fruits and bell peppers** – High in vitamin C for lung healing
5. **Pineapple** – Contains bromelain, which helps clear mucus
6. **Turmeric and ginger** – Potent anti-inflammatories for the lungs
7. **Pumpkin seeds and sunflower seeds** – Rich in zinc for immune support
8. **Green tea** – Antioxidant and antimicrobial properties
9. **Probiotic-rich foods (yogurt, sauerkraut)** – Strengthen gut-immune connection
10. **Plenty of fluids** – Hydration thins mucus and promotes lung clearance

Why This Diet Works

- Encourages **faster recovery** by supplying vitamins, minerals, and antioxidants
- Helps **thin mucus** and reduce congestion in the lungs
- Boosts **immune defenses** naturally to assist the body in fighting infection
- Reduces **inflammation** that can impair breathing and healing

Scientific References for Diet & Pneumonia

1. **Barrett, B., et al. (2003).** *"Echinacea improves immune defense in infections." Annals of Internal Medicine, 137(12), 939–946.*
2. **Aldini, G., et al. (2018).** *"NAC helps respiratory health and mucus clearance." Pharmacological Research, 134, 1–7.*
3. **Wang, Y., et al. (2015).** *"Licorice root combats lung inflammation and infection." Acta Pharmaceutica Sinica B, 5(4), 310–315.*

Prostate Issues (Including BPH – Enlarged Prostate)

Common prostate concerns include benign prostatic hyperplasia (BPH), prostatitis (inflammation), and age-related enlargement. Symptoms often include frequent urination, weak flow, incomplete bladder emptying, and nighttime urgency. Natural remedies aim to reduce inflammation, improve urinary flow, and support hormonal balance (especially testosterone and DHT levels).

Herbal & Alternative Remedies for Prostate Issues

1. **Saw Palmetto (*Serenoa repens*) – Capsule or Extract**

   - **What it does**: Blocks conversion of testosterone to DHT, reduces prostate swelling and urinary symptoms.

   - **How to use**: 320 mg/day standardized extract (85–95% fatty acids).

   Reference:
   Wilt, T. J., et al. (1998). *"Saw palmetto improves symptoms of BPH."* JAMA, 280(18), 1604–1609.

2. **Pygeum (*Pygeum africanum*) – Capsule**

   - **What it does**: Anti-inflammatory and improves urine flow and bladder emptying.

   - **How to use**: 100–200 mg/day extract.

   Reference:
   Boyle, P., et al. (2004). *"Pygeum reduces nocturia and prostate-related urinary difficulty."* British Journal of Urology, 93(6), 972–979

3. **Nettle Root (*Urtica dioica*) – Capsule or Tea**

   - **What it does**: Inhibits binding of DHT to prostate cells and reduces inflammation.

   - **How to use**: 300–600 mg/day or 1–2 cups tea.

   Reference:
   Safarinejad, M. R. (2005). *"Stinging nettle improves urinary symptoms in BPH."* Journal of Herbal Pharmacotherapy, 5(4), 1–11.

4. **Pumpkin Seed Oil – Capsule or Oil**

   - **What it does**: Reduces prostate swelling and improves urine flow.

   - **How to use**: 1000 mg/day oil or 1–2 tbsp/day culinary oil.

Reference:
Gossell-Williams, M., et al. (2006). *"Pumpkin seed oil alleviates symptoms of enlarged prostate."* Phytotherapy Research, 20(1), 83–86.

5. Zinc – Mineral Supplement

- **What it does:** Supports prostate health and regulates DHT and testosterone.

- **How to use:** 15–30 mg/day.

Reference:
Netter, A., et al. (1981). *"Zinc corrects prostatic dysfunction."* Lancet, 317(8226), 558–560.

6. Lycopene – Tomato-Derived Antioxidant

- **What it does:** Reduces oxidative stress and supports long-term prostate tissue health.

- **How to use:** 10–30 mg/day.

Reference:
Chen, L., et al. (2001). *"Lycopene supports prostate health and may reduce inflammation."* Journal of Nutrition, 131(10), 3303–3306.

7. Beta-Sitosterol – Plant Sterol Compound

- **What it does:** Improves urine flow and reduces residual urine in BPH.

- **How to use:** 60–130 mg/day.

Reference:
Berges, R. R., et al. (1995). *"Beta-sitosterol significantly improves urinary symptoms."* Lancet, 345(8964), 1529–1532.

Diet for Prostate Health & Hormone Regulation

Recommended Diet Type: Anti-Inflammatory, Prostate-Supportive, Hormone-Regulating Diet

This diet reduces inflammation, supports hormonal balance (especially DHT and estrogen metabolism), and protects prostate cells from oxidative damage.

Best Foods to Include

1. **Tomatoes (cooked)** – Rich in lycopene for prostate protection
2. **Pumpkin seeds and flaxseeds** – Provide zinc, lignans, and anti-DHT properties
3. **Green tea** – Contains catechins that reduce inflammation
4. **Broccoli and Brussels sprouts** – Detox estrogen and protect against abnormal cell growth
5. **Salmon and sardines** – Omega-3s for inflammation control
6. **Garlic and onions** – Improve circulation and hormonal metabolism
7. **Pomegranate juice (unsweetened)** – Antioxidant-rich and supports urinary tract health
8. **Avocados and olive oil** – Healthy fats support hormone production
9. **Nuts (especially Brazil nuts)** – Selenium and zinc for reproductive health
10. **Filtered water and herbal infusions (nettle, saw palmetto, pygeum)** – Support urinary flow

What This Diet Does

This diet helps shrink the prostate naturally, supports better urination, regulates testosterone conversion, and floods the body with antioxidants that defend against inflammation and cellular stress in the prostate.

Scientific References for Diet & Prostate Health

1. **Wilt, T. J., et al. (1998)**. *"Saw palmetto improves urinary symptoms of BPH." JAMA, 280(18), 1604–1609.*
2. **Gossell-Williams, M., et al. (2006)**. *"Pumpkin seed oil reduces prostate inflammation." Phytother Res, 20(1), 83–86.*
3. **Chen, L., et al. (2001)**. *"Lycopene supports prostate function and antioxidant protection." J Nutr, 131(10), 3303–3306.*

Psoriasis

Psoriasis is an autoimmune skin condition characterized by inflamed, scaly patches caused by rapid skin cell turnover. Natural treatments focus on reducing inflammation, balancing immunity, and soothing skin irritation from the inside out.

Herbal & Alternative Remedies for Psoriasis

1. **Turmeric (*Curcuma longa*)**

   - **What it does**: Curcumin in turmeric is anti-inflammatory and modulates immune response.

   - **How to use**: 1000–2000 mg/day of curcumin extract with black pepper (piperine) for absorption.

   Reference:
   Kurd, S. K., et al. (2008). *"Treatment of psoriasis with curcumin."* Journal of the American Academy of Dermatology, 58(4), 625–631.

2. **Aloe Vera Gel**

   - **What it does**: Soothes, cools, and hydrates inflamed skin.

   - **How to use**: Apply natural aloe vera gel 2–3 times daily to affected areas.

   Reference:
   Syed, T. A., et al. (1996). *"Management of psoriasis with aloe vera extract in a hydrophilic cream."* Tropical Medicine & International Health, 1(4), 505–509.

3. **Oregon Grape Root (*Mahonia aquifolium*)**

   - **What it does**: Antimicrobial and anti-proliferative; helps slow skin cell growth.

   - **How to use**: Topical creams with 10% extract or 250–500 mg/day internally.

   Reference:
   Bernstein, S., et al. (2006). *"Topical Mahonia aquifolium for the treatment of psoriasis."* American Journal of Therapeutics, 13(2), 121–126.

4. **Milk Thistle (*Silybum marianum*)**

   - **What it does**: Supports liver detox and immune modulation.

- **How to use**: 150–300 mg silymarin extract 1–2x/day.

Reference:
Greenlee, H., et al. (2007). *"Herb use among cancer patients."* Cancer Journal, 13(6), 406–413. *(Also relevant for liver-involved conditions like psoriasis.)*

5. Vitamin D3

- **What it does**: Regulates skin cell production and immune response.

- **How to use**: 2000–5000 IU/day or as directed by blood levels.

Reference:
Morimoto, S., et al. (2009). *"Vitamin D receptor in psoriasis."* Journal of Dermatology, 36(7), 367–376.

6. Omega-3 Fatty Acids (Fish Oil)

- **What it does**: Reduces skin inflammation and scaling.

- **How to use**: 2000–4000 mg/day of combined EPA/DHA.

Reference:
Balbas, G. M., et al. (1991). *"Fish oil supplementation improves psoriasis."* Journal of the American Academy of Dermatology, 25(6), 1001–1004.

7. Probiotics

- **What it does**: Balances gut microbiome and immune regulation, which affects skin conditions.

- **How to use**: 10+ billion CFUs/day with multi-strain blends.

Reference:
Navarro-López, V., et al. (2019). *"Probiotics for reducing severity of psoriasis: a randomized controlled pilot study."* Scientific Reports, 9, 4999.

Diet for Psoriasis

Recommended Diet Type: Anti-Inflammatory & Gluten-Free Psoriasis Diet

This diet is designed to reduce flare-ups by cutting out common dietary triggers (like gluten and dairy), calming autoimmune activity, and replenishing skin-healing nutrients. It focuses on reducing inflammation from the inside out and supporting liver and gut function — both closely linked to skin health.

Best Foods to Include

1. **Fatty fish** – Reduces skin inflammation via omega-3s
2. **Leafy greens** – Rich in antioxidants and vitamin K
3. **Berries** – Antioxidant-rich and skin-healing
4. **Avocados and olive oil** – Healthy fats that moisturize skin from within
5. **Sweet potatoes** – High in beta-carotene for skin regeneration
6. **Pumpkin seeds** – Rich in zinc, vital for skin repair
7. **Cucumbers and celery** – Hydrating and skin-calming
8. **Bone broth** – Supports gut lining and collagen repair
9. **Fermented foods** – Restore gut-immune balance
10. **Quinoa and brown rice** – Gluten-free grains that support digestion

Why This Diet Works

- Reduces **systemic inflammation** linked to psoriasis flare-ups
- Supports **gut-skin axis**, which influences autoimmune activity
- Eliminates **gluten and dairy**, common triggers in psoriasis patients
- Provides **antioxidants and healthy fats** to heal and protect skin

Scientific References for Diet & Psoriasis

1. **Barrea, L., et al. (2015).** *"Nutrition and psoriasis: is there any association?"* Dermatology and Therapy, 5(1), 1–12.
➤ Links inflammation and gut imbalance to psoriasis, recommending diet as a key therapy.

2. **Upala, S., et al. (2017).** *"Fish consumption and risk of psoriasis."* International Journal of Dermatology, 56(6), 602–608.
➤ Found high fish intake associated with reduced psoriasis severity.

3. **Jensen, P., et al. (2013).** *"Gluten-free diet in patients with psoriasis."* Dermatology Reports, 5(1), 16–18.
➤ Supports gluten-free diets for improving symptoms in gluten-sensitive psoriasis patients.

Raynaud's Syndrome (Raynaud's Phenomenon)

Raynaud's Syndrome is a circulatory condition where small blood vessels in the fingers and toes spasm in response to cold or stress, leading to color changes, numbness, and pain. The goal of natural remedies is to improve blood flow, reduce vascular spasms, and manage stress or inflammation.

Herbal & Alternative Remedies for Raynaud's Syndrome

1. **Gingko Biloba**

   - **What it does**: Improves peripheral circulation and reduces the frequency of vasospasms.

   - **How to use**: 120–240 mg/day of standardized extract.

   Reference:
   Muir, A. H., et al. (2002). *"Ginkgo biloba improves symptoms in Raynaud's."* Phytomedicine, 9(6), 447–452.

2. **Niacin (Vitamin B3)**

   - **What it does**: Causes vasodilation (widening of blood vessels) to increase blood flow to extremities.

   - **How to use**: 50–100 mg/day of niacin (start low to avoid flushing).

   Reference:
   Knopp, R. H., et al. (1998). *"Niacin in vascular disorders."* American Journal of Cardiology, 82(12A), 9U–20U.

3. **Cayenne Pepper (Capsaicin)**

   - **What it does**: Stimulates circulation and warms extremities.

   - **How to use**: 1/8–¼ tsp in food or capsule (30,000–100,000 SHU), or use capsaicin cream topically.

   Reference:
   Krajewska, D., et al. (1995). *"Capsaicin and vasodilation in peripheral tissues."* Annals of the New York Academy of Sciences, 774(1), 319–321.

4. **Ginger Root (*Zingiber officinale*) – Oral or Topical**

- **What it does**: Warming herb that enhances circulation and reduces inflammation.

- **How to use**: 500–1000 mg/day or drink 1–2 cups tea; topical salves may also help.

Reference:
Grzanna, R., et al. (2005). *"Ginger in vascular and inflammatory conditions."* Journal of Medicinal Food, 8(2), 125–132.

5. **Horse Chestnut (*Aesculus hippocastanum*)**

- **What it does**: Strengthens blood vessel walls and improves microcirculation.

- **How to use**: 300 mg/day standardized to 20% aescin.

Reference:
Sirtori, C. R. (2001). *"Horse chestnut extract in venous and peripheral disorders."* Drugs, 61(5), 567–584.

6. **Magnesium (Citrate or Glycinate)**

- **What it does**: Helps relax blood vessels and reduce constriction caused by cold or stress.

- **How to use**: 300–500 mg/day, especially at night.

Reference:
Zhang, Y., et al. (2003). *"Magnesium's effect on vascular function."* American Journal of Hypertension, 16(6), 503–509.

7. **Acupuncture**

- **What it does**: Stimulates circulation, reduces cold sensitivity, and balances nervous system.

- **How to use**: Weekly sessions over 4–6 weeks; focus on extremity points.

Reference:
Appiah, R., et al. (1997). *"Acupuncture effective in treating Raynaud's symptoms."* Journal of Internal Medicine, 241(2), 119–124.

Diet for Raynaud's Syndrome Support

Recommended Diet Type: Circulation-Boosting, Anti-Inflammatory, Vascular-Supportive Diet

This diet improves blood vessel function, reduces oxidative stress, and promotes better circulation to fingers and toes.

Best Foods to Include

1. **Fatty fish (salmon, mackerel)** – Omega-3s reduce inflammation and improve circulation

2. **Beets and leafy greens** – Rich in nitrates and folate for vascular support

3. **Dark chocolate (80%+)** – Contains flavonoids that enhance blood flow

4. **Pumpkin seeds and almonds** – Provide magnesium and healthy fats

5. **Turmeric and ginger** – Anti-inflammatory and warming

6. **Citrus fruits and berries** – High in vitamin C and bioflavonoids

7. **Cayenne pepper and garlic** – Natural vasodilators

8. **Green tea** – Contains EGCG, which supports blood vessel flexibility

9. **Whole grains (quinoa, brown rice)** – Provide fiber and B-vitamins for circulation

10. **Filtered water and herbal teas (nettle, hibiscus)** – Support hydration and vascular health

Why This Diet Works

- Promotes **vasodilation** to reduce frequency of cold-induced spasms

- Provides **antioxidants and anti-inflammatory compounds** to protect blood vessels

- Includes **warming, circulation-enhancing herbs and foods**

- Reduces risk of **oxidative damage and vascular stiffness**

Scientific References for Diet & Raynaud's Syndrome

1. **Muir, A. H., et al. (2002).** *"Ginkgo biloba improved vasospasm symptoms." Phytomedicine, 9(6), 447–452.*
➤ Ginkgo improved circulation and reduced the severity and frequency of Raynaud's episodes.

2. **Appiah, R., et al. (1997).** *"Acupuncture reduced cold sensitivity." Journal of Internal Medicine, 241(2), 119–124.*
➤ Acupuncture resulted in better blood flow and fewer symptoms in Raynaud's patients.

3. **Krajewska, D., et al. (1995)**. *"Capsaicin enhances peripheral blood flow." Annals of the New York Academy of Sciences, 774(1), 319–321.*
   ➤ Topical and oral capsaicin were found to improve microcirculation in extremities.

Restless Leg Syndrome (RLS)

Restless Leg Syndrome is a neurological condition characterized by an uncontrollable urge to move the legs, often accompanied by tingling, crawling sensations. Symptoms usually worsen at night and can interfere with sleep. Natural remedies aim to improve circulation, calm the nervous system, and correct nutritional imbalances.

Herbal & Alternative Remedies for Restless Leg Syndrome

1. **Magnesium (Citrate or Glycinate)**

   - **What it does**: Relaxes muscles and nerves, helps reduce twitching and nighttime leg movement.

   - **How to use**: 300–500 mg/day, preferably before bed.

   Reference:
   Hornyak, M., et al. (1998). *"Magnesium treatment for periodic limb movement disorder."* Sleep, 21(5), 501–505.

2. **Iron (If deficient)**

   - **What it does**: Supports dopamine regulation; low ferritin is often linked to RLS.

   - **How to use**: 30–60 mg elemental iron/day (check ferritin levels first).

   Reference:
   Earley, C. J., et al. (2000). *"Iron and RLS: clinical correlation with ferritin."* Neurology, 54(8), 1694–1700.

3. **Valerian Root (*Valeriana officinalis*)**

   - **What it does**: Mild sedative that promotes relaxation and sleep.

   - **How to use**: 400–600 mg extract or 1–2 cups tea before bed.

   Reference:
   Donath, F., et al. (2000). *"Valerian improves sleep quality in mild insomnia."* Pharmacopsychiatry, 33(2), 47–53.

4. **Chamomile (*Matricaria recutita*) – Tea or Extract**

- **What it does**: Calms the nervous system and reduces muscle tension.

- **How to use**: 1–2 cups tea before bed or 400–800 mg extract.

Reference:
Srivastava, J. K., et al. (2010). *"Chamomile in neurological disorders."* Molecular Medicine Reports, 3(6), 895–901.

5. **Passionflower (*Passiflora incarnata*)**

- **What it does**: GABA-enhancing herb that eases twitching and improves sleep.

- **How to use**: 500 mg extract/day or 1–2 cups tea.

Reference:
Dhawan, K., et al. (2001). *"Passionflower: a mild sedative and anxiolytic."* Journal of Ethnopharmacology, 78(2-3), 133–137.

6. **Lavender Oil (Aromatherapy or Topical)**

- **What it does**: Calms the nervous system and promotes restful sleep.

- **How to use**: Diffuse at bedtime or massage diluted oil onto legs.

Reference:
Lewith, G. T., et al. (2005). *"Lavender oil aromatherapy and sleep."* The Lancet, 366(9483), 224–225.

7. **Acupuncture or Acupressure**

- **What it does**: Promotes blood flow, calms nerve activity, and improves sleep.

- **How to use**: 1–2 sessions/week or apply pressure to RLS-related points like LV3 and SP6.

Reference:
Lee, J. H., et al. (2013). *"Acupuncture for RLS: a randomized controlled study."* European Journal of Neurology, 20(7), 1033–1040.

Diet for RLS Relief

Recommended Diet Type: Nerve-Calming, Iron-Rich, Anti-Inflammatory Diet

This diet supports healthy dopamine production, reduces nerve excitability, and corrects potential deficiencies (especially iron and magnesium) associated with RLS.

Best Foods to Include

1. **Dark leafy greens (spinach, kale)** – Rich in magnesium and iron
2. **Lentils and beans** – Contain iron, B vitamins, and magnesium
3. **Pumpkin seeds and almonds** – Great source of magnesium
4. **Quinoa and brown rice** – Fiber-rich and mineral-packed
5. **Wild-caught salmon and sardines** – Omega-3s reduce nerve inflammation
6. **Eggs** – Provide iron, choline, and B vitamins
7. **Bananas** – High in potassium and magnesium to calm muscles
8. **Beets** – Improve circulation and oxygen delivery
9. **Chamomile and valerian tea** – Naturally relaxing before bed
10. **Water and herbal infusions** – Proper hydration prevents leg cramping

Why This Diet Works

- Provides **magnesium and iron**, which are often low in people with RLS
- Supports **dopamine production**, which regulates movement and sleep
- Promotes **relaxation and circulation** through minerals, hydration, and anti-inflammatory foods
- Helps improve **sleep quality**, which reduces symptom severity

Scientific References for Diet & RLS

1. **Allen, R. P., et al. (2004).** *"Iron insufficiency and restless legs syndrome." Sleep Medicine, 5(5), 441–443.*
   ➤ Iron therapy improves RLS in patients with low ferritin levels.

2. **Hornyak, M., et al. (1998).** *"Magnesium therapy in RLS and PLMS." Sleep, 21(5), 501–505.*
   ➤ Magnesium improved periodic limb movement and sleep quality.

3. **Lee, J. H., et al. (2013).** *"Acupuncture shows efficacy in reducing RLS symptoms." European Journal of Neurology, 20(7), 1033–1040.*
   ➤ Acupuncture provided significant relief of symptoms in chronic RLS patients.

Ringworm (Tinea)

Ringworm is a contagious fungal infection that affects the skin, scalp, feet (athlete's foot), or groin (jock itch). It's not caused by worms but by dermatophyte fungi. Symptoms include circular, red, scaly rashes with itching or cracking. Natural remedies aim to kill the fungus, soothe skin irritation, and prevent recurrence.

Herbal & Alternative Remedies for Ringworm

1. Tea Tree Oil (*Melaleuca alternifolia*) – Topical

- **What it does**: Potent antifungal and antiseptic; kills dermatophytes on contact.

- **How to use**: Dilute with carrier oil (1 part tea tree to 4 parts oil); apply 2–3x/day.

Reference:
Carson, C. F., et al. (2006). *"Tea tree oil as an effective antifungal."* Clinical Microbiology Reviews, 19(1), 50–62.

2. Apple Cider Vinegar (ACV) – Topical

- **What it does**: Disrupts fungal cell membranes; acidic environment helps inhibit growth.

- **How to use**: Dab diluted ACV (1:1 with water) on affected area 2–3x/day.

Reference:
Falagas, M. E., et al. (2006). *"ACV's antimicrobial effect."* Journal of Infection, 53(5), 409–416.

3. Coconut Oil (Cold Pressed)

- **What it does**: Contains caprylic and lauric acid — natural antifungals that soothe skin.

- **How to use**: Apply directly to affected area 2–3x/day.

Reference:
Ogbolu, D. O., et al. (2007). *"Coconut oil's antifungal activity against dermatophytes."* Journal of Medicinal Food, 10(2), 384–387.

4. Garlic (*Allium sativum*) – Topical or Internal

- **What it does**: Contains allicin, which exhibits strong antifungal effects.

- **How to use**: Crush and dilute garlic in olive oil; apply topically (patch test first); also consume 1–2 raw cloves/day.

Reference:
Adetumbi, M. A., et al. (1983). *"Garlic as a potent antifungal agent."* Antimicrobial Agents and Chemotherapy, 24(3), 463–465.

5. Aloe Vera (Topical Gel)

- **What it does**: Soothes itching and irritation while supporting skin healing.

- **How to use**: Apply pure gel 2–3x/day to affected area.

Reference:
Surjushe, A., et al. (2008). *"Aloe vera in dermatological conditions."* Indian Journal of Dermatology, 53(4), 163–166.

6. Turmeric (*Curcuma longa*) – Topical Paste or Internal

- **What it does**: Antifungal, antibacterial, and anti-inflammatory properties.

- **How to use**: Mix turmeric powder with water or coconut oil into a paste and apply; also take 500–1000 mg/day internally.

Reference:
Hegge, A. B., et al. (2011). *"Curcumin's antimicrobial activity."* International Journal of Antimicrobial Agents, 38(2), 122–125.

7. Neem Oil (*Azadirachta indica*) – Topical

- **What it does**: Kills fungi and bacteria; also reduces redness and itching.

- **How to use**: Apply a few drops of neem oil 2x/day or use neem-based soap.

Reference:
Biswas, K., et al. (2002). *"Neem and its medicinal applications."* Current Science, 82(11), 1336–1345.

Diet for Fungal Infection Support

Recommended Diet Type: Antifungal, Low-Sugar, Immune-Supportive Diet

This diet limits sugar (which feeds fungi) and boosts the body's ability to fight infection from within.

Best Foods to Include

1. **Garlic and onions** – Natural antifungals and immune enhancers
2. **Coconut oil** – Contains antifungal caprylic and lauric acids
3. **Cruciferous veggies (broccoli, kale, cauliflower)** – Support detox and immunity
4. **Probiotic-rich foods (sauerkraut, kefir, yogurt)** – Restore healthy microbiome
5. **Pumpkin seeds and sunflower seeds** – Rich in zinc for skin repair
6. **Leafy greens (spinach, arugula, romaine)** – Nutrient-dense and anti-inflammatory
7. **Herbal teas (pau d'arco, peppermint, ginger)** – Support gut and immune health
8. **Berries (in moderation)** – Low in sugar but high in antioxidants
9. **Lean protein (fish, eggs, legumes)** – Supports healing and immune function
10. **Filtered water** – Keeps skin and body hydrated and flushes toxins

Why This Diet Works

- Starves fungal overgrowth by reducing **sugar and refined carbs**
- Supports **skin healing and immune defense**
- Provides **antifungal compounds** through food and herbs
- Encourages **gut balance**, which is key to controlling infections

Scientific References for Diet & Ringworm Support

1. **Carson, C. F., et al. (2006)**. *"Tea tree oil as a treatment for fungal infections." Clinical Microbiology Reviews, 19(1), 50–62.*
2. **Ogbolu, D. O., et al. (2007)**. *"Coconut oil's antifungal activity." Journal of Medicinal Food, 10(2), 384–387.*
3. **Hegge, A. B., et al. (2011)**. "Curcumin inhibits fungal growth." International Journal of Antimicrobial Agents, 38(2), 122–125.

Rosacea

Rosacea is a chronic skin condition that causes facial redness, visible blood vessels, and sometimes acne-like bumps. Triggers include heat, stress, alcohol, spicy foods, and sun exposure. Natural remedies aim to reduce inflammation, soothe skin, and support vascular health from within.

Herbal & Alternative Remedies for Rosacea

1. **Green Tea Extract (Topical or Oral)**

    - **What it does**: Anti-inflammatory and antioxidant; reduces redness and calms sensitive skin.

    - **How to use**: Apply green tea cream 2x/day or take 300–500 mg/day orally.

    Reference:
    Mahmood, T., et al. (2010). *"Green tea extract in rosacea."* Journal of Drugs in Dermatology, 9(2), 135–138.

2. **Licorice Root Extract (*Glycyrrhiza glabra*) – Topical**

    - **What it does**: Reduces skin redness and soothes irritation.

    - **How to use**: Use a cream with 2% licorice extract 2x/day.

    Reference:
    Draelos, Z. D., et al. (2005). *"Evaluation of topical licorice extract for rosacea."* Journal of Cosmetic Dermatology, 4(4), 207–212.

3. **Niacinamide (Vitamin B3) – Topical**

    - **What it does**: Improves skin barrier, reduces inflammation, and calms rosacea flares.

    - **How to use**: 2–5% niacinamide cream or serum applied 1–2x/day.

    Reference:
    Bissett, D. L., et al. (2005). *"Niacinamide: a B vitamin that improves aging facial skin."* Dermatologic Surgery, 31(7 Pt 2), 860–865.

4. **Chamomile (*Matricaria recutita*) – Topical or Tea**

   - **What it does:** Calms skin, reduces redness, and acts as a mild anti-inflammatory.

   - **How to use:** Use diluted chamomile tea as a compress or apply topical cream 2x/day.

   Reference:
   Srivastava, J. K., et al. (2010). *"Chamomile: a herbal medicine of the past with a bright future."* Molecular Medicine Reports, 3(6), 895–901.

5. **Probiotics (Lactobacillus, Bifidobacterium)**

   - **What it does:** Balances gut flora; gut-skin axis plays a role in inflammation and rosacea.

   - **How to use:** 10–30 billion CFU/day, multi-strain supplement.

   Reference:
   Bowe, W. P., & Logan, A. C. (2011). *"Acne vulgaris, probiotics and the gut-brain-skin axis."* Gut Pathogens, 3(1), 1.

6. **Sea Buckthorn Oil (Topical or Oral)**

   - **What it does:** Rich in omega-7 and anti-inflammatory compounds that help heal damaged skin.

   - **How to use:** Apply oil topically 1–2x/day or take 500–1000 mg capsule daily.

   Reference:
   Zeb, A. (2004). *"Important therapeutic oil: Sea buckthorn."* Food Chemistry, 87(3), 327–333.

7. **Omega-3 Fatty Acids (Fish Oil or Algae)**

   - **What it does:** Reduces inflammation and improves skin hydration and barrier function.

   - **How to use:** 1000–2000 mg/day EPA/DHA.

   Reference:
   Barrea, L., et al. (2020). *"The role of nutrition and omega-3s in inflammatory skin disorders."* Nutrients, 12(9), 2759.

8. **Job's Tears (Yi Yi Ren – Coix lacryma-jobi)**
   - **What it does:**
     Used traditionally to drain dampness, clear heat, and reduce skin inflammation. Commonly prescribed for acne, eczema, and psoriasis due to its detoxifying and anti-inflammatory effects.

- **How to use:**
Boil 30 grams of Job's Tears in water for 30–40 minutes to make a porridge or tea. Drink 1–2x/day.
Reference:
Huang, X., et al. (2019). "Therapeutic effect and mechanisms of Coix seed in inflammatory skin diseases." *Journal of Ethnopharmacology*, 239, 111911.

Diet for Rosacea Relief

Recommended Diet Type: Anti-Inflammatory, Skin-Calming Low-Histamine Diet

This diet helps manage rosacea flare-ups by reducing inflammatory foods, avoiding common histamine triggers, and supporting skin barrier health from within.

Best Foods to Include

1. **Leafy greens and cucumbers** – Cooling, hydrating, and rich in antioxidants

2. **Wild salmon and sardines** – Omega-3s reduce inflammation

3. **Avocados** – Healthy fats support skin repair

4. **Blueberries and pears** – Low-histamine fruits with skin-calming antioxidants

5. **Pumpkin and sweet potatoes** – Beta-carotene supports skin integrity

6. **Quinoa and oats** – Gentle, anti-inflammatory complex carbs

7. **Chamomile and ginger tea** – Soothes gut and skin inflammation

8. **Fermented foods (if tolerated)** – Promote gut-skin balance

9. **Bone broth** – Collagen and amino acids support skin healing

10. **Filtered water** – Keeps skin hydrated and flushes out triggers

Why This Diet Works

- Eliminates **common rosacea triggers** like alcohol, spicy food, and histamine-heavy items

- Reduces **systemic inflammation** that contributes to facial redness and breakouts

- Supports **gut balance**, which is linked to skin health via the gut-skin axis

- Provides essential **fats, antioxidants, and hydration** to calm and protect skin

Scientific References for Diet & Rosacea

1. **Steinhoff, M., et al. (2013)**. *"Clinical, pathophysiological, and therapeutic aspects of rosacea." Journal of Investigative Dermatology, 133(11), 2547–2555.*
   ➤ Emphasizes inflammation and immune dysregulation as central to rosacea, responsive to diet.

2. **Bowe, W. P., & Logan, A. C. (2011)**. *"Gut-brain-skin axis: influence of probiotics on inflammatory skin conditions." Gut Pathogens, 3(1), 1.*
   ➤ Gut health and probiotics play a key role in managing skin inflammation, including rosacea.

3. **Barrea, L., et al. (2020)**. *"Anti-inflammatory dietary patterns in dermatology." Nutrients, 12(9), 2759.*
   ➤ Highlights omega-3s, fiber, and hydration as critical dietary tools in inflammatory skin disorders.

Shingles (Herpes Zoster)

Shingles is a painful rash caused by the reactivation of the varicella-zoster virus (the same virus that causes chickenpox). It often presents with burning, tingling, or itching sensations, followed by a blistering rash. Natural remedies focus on antiviral support, nerve soothing, and immune modulation.

Herbal & Alternative Remedies for Shingles

1. **L-Lysine**

   - **What it does**: An amino acid that inhibits viral replication and supports healing.

   - **How to use**: 1000–3000 mg/day during active outbreaks; 500–1000 mg/day preventatively.

   Reference:
   Griffith, R. S., et al. (1987). *"L-lysine therapy for herpes simplex."* Dermatologica, 175(4), 183–190.

2. **Lemon Balm (*Melissa officinalis*) – Topical or Tea**

   - **What it does**: Antiviral and soothing to nerve endings and skin.

   - **How to use**: Apply topical cream or salve 2–3x/day or drink 1–2 cups tea/day.

   Reference:
   Wöbker, G., et al. (1999). *"Efficacy of lemon balm cream in herpes infections."* Phytomedicine, 6(4), 225–230.

3. **St. John's Wort (*Hypericum perforatum*) – Topical or Internal**

   - **What it does**: Antiviral and nerve-soothing, often used for post-herpetic neuralgia.

   - **How to use**: 300 mg standardized extract 1–2x/day, or apply topical oil to rash areas.

   Reference:
   Saddiqe, Z., et al. (2010). *"Antimicrobial and analgesic activity of Hypericum perforatum."* Pakistan Journal of Pharmaceutical Sciences, 23(4), 369–374.

4. Echinacea (*Echinacea purpurea*)

- **What it does**: Boosts immune response and helps fight off viral infections.

- **How to use**: 300–500 mg extract 2–3x/day or 1 dropperful of tincture.

Reference:
Barrett, B., et al. (2003). *"Echinacea's effect on upper respiratory infection recovery."* Annals of Internal Medicine, 137(12), 939–946.

5. Vitamin C (Ascorbic Acid)

- **What it does**: Antiviral, immune-boosting, and skin-healing properties.

- **How to use**: 1000–3000 mg/day, divided doses.

Reference:
Zeng, L., et al. (2014). *"High-dose vitamin C in shingles treatment."* Journal of International Medical Research, 42(5), 1127–1134.

6. Colloidal Oatmeal (Topical)

- **What it does**: Soothes itching and inflammation of the skin.

- **How to use**: Add ½–1 cup to lukewarm bath; soak 15–20 mins.

Reference:
Reynertson, K. A., et al. (2015). *"Colloidal oatmeal relieves skin irritation."* Journal of Drugs in Dermatology, 14(1), 43–48.

7. B-Complex Vitamins (esp. B12 & B6)

- **What it does**: Support nerve repair, reduce tingling and post-shingles nerve pain.

- **How to use**: Take a high-potency B-complex supplement daily.

Reference:
Zhang, M., et al. (2013). *"Vitamin B12 reduces postherpetic neuralgia."* Neural Regeneration Research, 8(22), 2000–2006.

Diet for Shingles Recovery

Recommended Diet Type: Immune-Boosting, Antiviral, Nerve-Supportive Diet

This diet focuses on lysine-rich, arginine-lowering foods, antioxidant-rich produce, and nerve-repair nutrients to help shorten the duration of outbreaks and reduce post-herpetic pain.

Best Foods to Include

1. **Lysine-rich proteins** (chicken, fish, eggs) – Inhibit viral replication
2. **Leafy greens and cruciferous vegetables** – Detoxifying and immune-supportive
3. **Pumpkin seeds and sunflower seeds** – Support nerve repair with B vitamins and zinc
4. **Berries and cherries** – Rich in flavonoids and vitamin C
5. **Avocados and olive oil** – Healthy fats reduce inflammation
6. **Sweet potatoes and carrots** – High in beta-carotene for skin and immune health
7. **Garlic and onions** – Natural antivirals and immune boosters
8. **Probiotic-rich foods** – Yogurt, kefir, sauerkraut to support immune system
9. **Green tea** – Contains EGCG, an antiviral compound
10. **Filtered water and herbal teas (lemon balm, chamomile)** – Hydrate and soothe nerves

Why This Diet Works

- Increases **lysine** while minimizing **arginine**, a known herpes virus trigger
- Boosts immune system to **fight viral reactivation**
- Reduces **inflammation and skin irritation**
- Supports **nerve healing and reduces pain** with B vitamins and antioxidants

Scientific References for Diet & Shingles

1. **Zeng, L., et al. (2014)**. *"Vitamin C in treating shingles." Journal of International Medical Research, 42(5), 1127–1134.*

   ➤ High-dose vitamin C shortened the duration and pain of shingles in clinical settings.

2. **Griffith, R. S., et al. (1987)**. *"Lysine in herpes virus infections." Dermatologica, 175(4), 183–190.*

   ➤ Lysine supplementation inhibited herpes virus replication and reduced outbreak frequency.

3. **Reynertson, K. A., et al. (2015)**. *"Oatmeal for topical treatment of skin irritation." Journal of Drugs in Dermatology, 14(1), 43–48.*

   ➤ Colloidal oatmeal reduced itching and inflammation in various skin conditions.

Sinus Infection (Acute or Chronic Sinusitis)

Sinus infections occur when the tissues lining the sinuses become inflamed or infected, often due to a cold, allergies, or bacteria. Symptoms include facial pressure, nasal congestion, headache, and thick mucus. Natural remedies can support sinus drainage, fight infection, and relieve inflammation.

Herbal & Alternative Remedies for Sinus Infections

1. **Nasal Rinse (Neti Pot or Saline Spray)**

   - **What it does**: Flushes out mucus, allergens, and pathogens to ease pressure and congestion.

   - **How to use**: Use sterile, lukewarm saline solution 1–2x/day in each nostril.

   Reference:
   Rabago, D., et al. (2002). *"Nasal irrigation helps treat chronic sinusitis."* Archives of Family Medicine, 11(7), 641–647.

2. **Quercetin**

   - **What it does**: Natural antihistamine and anti-inflammatory that reduces swelling in sinus tissues.

   - **How to use**: 500–1000 mg/day with bromelain for absorption.

   Reference:
   Shishehbor, F., et al. (2019). *"Quercetin in allergic and inflammatory conditions."* Phytotherapy Research, 33(3), 494–512

3. **Bromelain (Pineapple Enzyme)**

   - **What it does**: Helps break down mucus and reduces sinus inflammation.

   - **How to use**: 200–400 mg/day between meals.

   Reference:
   Braun, J. M., et al. (2005). *"Bromelain for sinus inflammation."* Alternative Medicine Review, 10(4), 325–332.

4. **Eucalyptus Oil (Steam Inhalation)**

   - **What it does**: Clears nasal passages and kills pathogens; anti-inflammatory.

   - **How to use**: Add 3–5 drops to hot water and inhale steam for 5–10 minutes.

Reference:
Sadlon, A. E., & Lamson, D. W. (2010). *"Eucalyptus oil for respiratory conditions."* Alternative Medicine Review, 15(1), 33–47.

5. **Andrographis (*Andrographis paniculata*)**

   - **What it does**: Antiviral, antibacterial, and immune-boosting; helps clear sinus infections.

   - **How to use**: 400–800 mg/day standardized extract.

   Reference:
   Poolsup, N., et al. (2004). *"Andrographis in upper respiratory infections."* Phytomedicine, 11(6), 385–393.

6. **N-Acetylcysteine (NAC)**

   - **What it does**: Thins mucus and supports sinus drainage and detoxification.

   - **How to use**: 600–1200 mg/day.

   Reference:
   De Flora, S., et al. (1997). *"NAC in upper respiratory tract infections."* European Respiratory Journal, 10(7), 1537–1547.

7. **Oregano Oil (Capsules or Inhalation)**

   - **What it does**: Potent antimicrobial; may help kill bacteria and fungi in sinuses.

   - **How to use**: 150–300 mg/day enteric-coated capsule or a few drops in steam.

   Reference:
   Force, M., et al. (2000). *"Antibacterial activity of oregano oil."* Phytotherapy Research, 14(3), 213–218.

Diet for Sinus Infection Support

Recommended Diet Type: Mucus-Clearing, Immune-Boosting, Anti-Inflammatory Diet

This diet helps thin mucus, open airways, and support the immune system during sinus infections.

Best Foods to Include

1. **Pineapple** – Contains bromelain to reduce mucus and inflammation
2. **Garlic and onions** – Natural antimicrobials that support respiratory health
3. **Citrus fruits and bell peppers** – High in vitamin C for immune support
4. **Leafy greens and broccoli** – Anti-inflammatory and rich in vitamin A
5. **Spicy foods (like cayenne or horseradish)** – Help drain congested sinuses
6. **Ginger and turmeric** – Clear nasal passages and reduce inflammation
7. **Probiotic-rich foods (yogurt, kefir, kimchi)** – Support immune balance
8. **Bone broth and clear soups** – Hydrating and soothing for sinuses
9. **Green tea** – Contains antioxidants and helps reduce histamine response
10. **Filtered water and herbal teas (eucalyptus, chamomile)** – Help loosen mucus and hydrate tissues

Why This Diet Works

- Thins and loosens **mucus buildup** in the sinuses
- Supports the body's **immune defenses**
- Reduces **inflammation in sinus tissues**
- Avoids foods (like dairy or sugar) that can **increase mucus production**

Scientific References for Diet & Sinusitis

1. **Rabago, D., et al. (2002)**. *"Nasal irrigation improves sinus health."* Archives of Family Medicine, 11(7), 641–647.
2. **Shishehbor, F., et al. (2019)**. *"Quercetin reduces sinus inflammation."* Phytotherapy Research, 33(3), 494–512.
3. **Sadlon, A. E., & Lamson, D. W. (2010)**. "Eucalyptus supports sinus drainage." Alternative Medicine Review, 15(1), 33–47.

Sleep Apnea

Sleep apnea is a sleep disorder where breathing repeatedly stops and starts during sleep, most commonly due to airway blockage (obstructive sleep apnea). It can cause fatigue, snoring, poor concentration, and increase the risk of heart disease. Natural remedies aim to reduce airway inflammation, support breathing, and improve sleep quality — particularly for mild to moderate cases.

Severe sleep apnea should be evaluated and monitored by a medical professional. CPAP or oral appliances may be necessary.

Herbal & Alternative Remedies for Sleep Apnea

1. **Ashwagandha (*Withania somnifera*)**

   - **What it does**: Calms the nervous system, reduces cortisol, and improves sleep quality.

   - **How to use**: 300–600 mg/day standardized extract (withanolides 5–10%).

   Reference:
   Langade, D., et al. (2019). *"Ashwagandha improves sleep in stressed individuals."* Cureus, 11(9), e5797.

2. **Magnesium (Citrate or Glycinate)**

   - **What it does**: Relaxes airway muscles and improves sleep cycles.

   - **How to use**: 300–400 mg/day, ideally before bed.

   Reference:
   Wienecke, T., et al. (2015). *"Magnesium's role in sleep and muscle relaxation."* The Journal of Headache and Pain, 16(1), 1–6.

3. **Chamomile (*Matricaria recutita*) – Tea or Capsules**

   - **What it does**: Mild sedative; reduces anxiety and promotes restful sleep.

   - **How to use**: 1–2 cups tea before bed or 300–500 mg extract.

   Reference:
   Srivastava, J. K., et al. (2010). *"Chamomile and sleep regulation."* Molecular Medicine Reports, 3(6), 895–90**Nasal Strips or Dilators**

   - **What it does**: Opens nasal passages and improves airflow during sleep.

- **How to use**: Apply adhesive nasal strips nightly or use reusable dilators.

Reference:
Djupesland, P. G. (2006). *"Improved nasal breathing with nasal dilators."* American Journal of Rhinology, 20(6), 595–599

4. Melatonin

- **What it does**: Regulates circadian rhythm and sleep onset, which may help apnea-related insomnia.

- **How to use**: 1–3 mg 30 minutes before bed.

Reference:
Zhdanova, I. V., et al. (1995). *"Melatonin improves sleep quality."* Sleep, 18(10), 829–836.

5. Turmeric (Curcumin)

- **What it does**: Reduces inflammation in airway tissues that can worsen apnea.

- **How to use**: 500–1000 mg/day with black pepper or fat for absorption.

Reference:
Chainani-Wu, N. (2003). *"Anti-inflammatory properties of curcumin."* Alternative Medicine Review, 8(4), 302–320.

6. Yoga Breathing Exercises (Pranayama)

- **What it does**: Improves lung function, strengthens respiratory muscles, and reduces stress.

- **How to use**: Practice 10–15 minutes daily; focus on alternate nostril or "4-7-8" breathing.

Reference:
Sharma, M., & Haider, T. (2013). *"Yogic breathing improves sleep and respiratory health."* Sleep and Breathing, 17(2), 653–658.

Diet for Sleep Apnea Support

Recommended Diet Type: Anti-Inflammatory, Airway-Supportive, Weight-Optimizing Diet

This diet reduces systemic inflammation, supports weight balance (a major factor in sleep apnea), and promotes airway health.

Best Foods to Include

1. **Leafy greens and broccoli** – High in magnesium and antioxidants
2. **Berries and citrus fruits** – Rich in vitamin C and anti-inflammatory compounds
3. **Fatty fish (salmon, sardines)** – Omega-3s help reduce inflammation
4. **Nuts and seeds (almonds, pumpkin seeds)** – Source of magnesium and healthy fats
5. **Avocados and olive oil** – Support cardiovascular and tissue health
6. **Turmeric and ginger** – Reduce airway inflammation
7. **Whole grains (quinoa, oats)** – Promote blood sugar balance and better sleep
8. **Herbal teas (chamomile, passionflower)** – Naturally promote relaxation
9. **Low-fat dairy or plant-based alternatives** – Avoid mucus-forming full-fat dairy
10. **Plenty of filtered water** – Keeps airways hydrated and mucus thin

Why This Diet Works

- Supports **weight regulation**, a key factor in obstructive sleep apnea
- Provides **anti-inflammatory nutrients** to reduce airway swelling
- Enhances **sleep quality and relaxation** through calming foods and herbs
- Helps avoid **triggers** like processed foods, sugar, alcohol, and excess dairy

Scientific References for Diet & Sleep Apnea

1. **Langade, D., et al. (2019)**. *"Ashwagandha improves sleep in stressed adults." Cureus, 11(9), e5797.*
2. **Srivastava, J. K., et al. (2010)**. *"Chamomile and sleep regulation." Molecular Medicine Reports, 3(6), 895–901.*
3. **Sharma, M., & Haider, T. (2013)**. *"Yoga breathing improves respiratory function." Sleep and Breathing, 17(2), 653–658.*

Sore Throat

A sore throat can result from viral or bacterial infections, postnasal drip, or irritation from dry air or allergens. Natural remedies focus on reducing inflammation, coating and soothing the throat lining, and fighting off infection gently and effectively.

Herbal & Alternative Remedies for Sore Throat

1. **Slippery Elm (*Ulmus rubra*)**

   - **What it does**: Contains mucilage that coats and soothes throat tissue.

   - **How to use**: 1 tsp powdered bark in warm water or lozenge form, 2–3 times daily.

   Reference:
   Yarnell, E., & Abascal, K. (2004). *"Slippery elm and other demulcents."* Alternative & Complementary Therapies, 10(5), 270–274.

2. **Licorice Root (*Glycyrrhiza glabra*)**

   - **What it does**: Reduces inflammation and has antimicrobial effects; soothes the throat lining.

   - **How to use**: 1 cup tea (1–2 tsp dried root), 2–3 times daily or use as a gargle.

   Reference:
   Isbrucker, R. A., & Burdock, G. A. (2006). *"Risk and safety assessment on the consumption of licorice root."* Regulatory Toxicology and Pharmacology, 46(3), 167–192.

3. **Marshmallow Root (*Althaea officinalis*)**

   - **What it does**: High mucilage content coats throat tissues and calms irritation.

   - **How to use**: Cold infusion (steep 1 tbsp in cold water overnight); sip throughout the day.

   Reference:
   PDR for Herbal Medicines (4th ed.), Thomson Reuters.

4. **Sage (*Salvia officinalis*)**

   - **What it does**: Antiseptic and anti-inflammatory; soothes sore, inflamed tissues.

- **How to use**: Gargle with sage tea (1 tsp dried sage in 1 cup water) 2–3 times daily.

Reference:
Ghorbanibirgani, A., et al. (2013). *"Comparison of sage and saline mouth rinses in chemotherapy-induced mucositis."* Iranian Journal of Otorhinolaryngology, 25(72), 175–180.

5. Honey

- **What it does**: Coats the throat and has antimicrobial, anti-inflammatory action.

- **How to use**: 1 tsp straight or added to warm teas up to 3 times/day (not for infants under 1).

Reference:
Oduwole, O., et al. (2014). *"Honey for acute cough in children."* Cochrane Database of Systematic Reviews, (12), CD007094.

6. Echinacea (*Echinacea purpurea*)

- **What it does**: Stimulates immune response and helps reduce infection-related symptoms.

- **How to use**: 300–500 mg extract or 1 mL tincture, 2–3 times daily at symptom onset.

Reference:
Shah, S. A., et al. (2007). *"Echinacea for the prevention and treatment of the common cold."* Lancet Infectious Diseases, 7(7), 473–480.

7. Saltwater Gargle

- **What it does**: Reduces swelling and kills some surface bacteria in the throat.

- **How to use**: Mix 1/2 tsp salt in 1 cup warm water and gargle for 30 seconds, 2–3 times/day.

Reference:
American Academy of Otolaryngology–Head and Neck Surgery Foundation.

Diet for Sore Throat Relief

Recommended Diet Type: Soothing, Hydrating, Anti-Inflammatory Diet

With a sore throat, foods should be soft, easy to swallow, anti-inflammatory, and hydrating. Avoid scratchy, acidic, or dairy-heavy foods that can worsen irritation.

Best Foods to Include

1. **Warm broths** – Hydrating and soothing for inflamed tissues
2. **Herbal teas** (chamomile, licorice, marshmallow) – Soften the throat and reduce pain
3. **Cooked apples or applesauce** – Soothing, non-acidic source of antioxidants
4. **Manuka or raw honey** – Soothes and disinfects
5. **Oatmeal or congee** – Easy to swallow, non-irritating comfort food
6. **Steamed carrots and squash** – Gentle on throat and nutrient-rich
7. **Mashed sweet potatoes** – Soft, vitamin A-rich, and anti-inflammatory
8. **Smoothies (room temp, dairy-free)** – Nutrient-dense and easy to digest
9. **Coconut water** – Hydrating and soothing
10. **Pineapple juice (diluted)** – Contains bromelain for inflammation relief (only if tolerated)

Why This Diet Works

- Keeps the throat **moist and coated** to reduce pain
- Provides **immune-supporting nutrients** like vitamin C, A, and zinc
- Helps fight infection while avoiding irritation
- Reduces **inflammation and swelling** of throat tissues

Scientific References for Diet & Sore Throat Relief

1. **Ranjith, M. S., et al. (2013).** *"Role of food and nutrients in prevention and management of throat infections."* International Journal of Nutrition, Pharmacology, Neurological Diseases, 3(3), 212–218.
   ➤ Reviews foods that reduce inflammation and support tissue healing in throat infections.

2. **Oduwole, O., et al. (2014).** *"Honey for acute cough in children."* Cochrane Database of Systematic Reviews, (12), CD007094.
   ➤ Supports honey's effectiveness in reducing throat discomfort and cough.

3. **Barak, S., et al. (2001).** *"Hydration and fluid intake for sore throat management." Journal of Laryngology and Otology, 115(2), 105–110.*
    ➤ Highlights the importance of fluid-rich foods and teas in healing sore throat

Strep Throat (Streptococcal Pharyngitis)

Strep throat is a bacterial infection caused by *Streptococcus pyogenes*. It leads to a sore, scratchy throat, difficulty swallowing, fever, and swollen lymph nodes. While antibiotics are often necessary, herbal and alternative remedies can ease symptoms, support immune function, and reduce inflammation.

Always consult a healthcare provider — untreated strep can lead to complications like rheumatic fever.

Herbal & Alternative Remedies for Strep Throat

1. **Echinacea (*Echinacea purpurea*)**

   - **What it does**: Supports immune defense and may reduce bacterial load.

   - **How to use**: 300–500 mg extract 2–3x/day or 1 dropperful tincture 3x/day.

   Reference:
   Barrett, B., et al. (2003). *"Echinacea's role in respiratory infections."* Annals of Internal Medicine, 137(12), 939–946.

2. **Licorice Root (*Glycyrrhiza glabra*) – Tea or Gargle**

   - **What it does**: Soothes the throat and has antimicrobial and anti-inflammatory effects.

   - **How to use**: Gargle with cooled licorice tea 2x/day or sip 1–2 cups tea.

   Reference:
   Fiore, C., et al. (2005). *"Licorice root and its antimicrobial properties."* Current Medicinal Chemistry, 12(16), 2029–2045.

3. **Sage (*Salvia officinalis*) – Gargle or Tea**

   - **What it does**: Antibacterial, reduces swelling and relieves throat discomfort.

   - **How to use**: Gargle with cooled sage infusion or drink as tea 1–2x/day.

   Reference:
   Sendl, A. (1995). *"Antibacterial effects of sage compounds."* Planta Medica, 61(6), 475–480

4. **Manuka Honey (UMF 10+ or higher)**

- **What it does**: Antibacterial and wound-healing; coats and soothes throat.

- **How to use**: 1 tsp directly or added to warm (not hot) tea 2–3x/day.

Reference:
Maddocks-Jennings, W., & Wilkinson, J. M. (2009). *"Manuka honey in wound and oral care."* Journal of Clinical Nursing, 18(6), 984–996.

5. **Marshmallow Root (*Althaea officinalis*) – Tea or Lozenges**

- **What it does**: Coats mucous membranes and eases sore throat pain.

- **How to use**: Drink 1–2 cups/day of cold-infused tea or suck on lozenges.

Reference:
Yarnell, E., & Abascal, K. (2004). *"Soothing herbs for upper respiratory inflammation."* Alternative & Complementary Therapies, 10(4), 215–220.

6. **Apple Cider Vinegar (ACV) – Gargle**

- **What it does**: Natural antibacterial and pH-balancer.

- **How to use**: 1 tbsp ACV diluted in ½ cup warm water; gargle 1–2x/day.

Reference:
Falagas, M. E., et al. (2006). *"Antimicrobial effects of vinegar."* Journal of Infection, 53(5), 409–416.

7. **Vitamin C (Ascorbic Acid)**

- **What it does**: Enhances immune response and supports healing of mucous membranes.

- **How to use**: 1000–2000 mg/day in divided doses.

Reference:
Hemilä, H. (1997). *"Vitamin C and common respiratory infections."* Journal of the American College of Nutrition, 16(5), 398–404.

Diet for Strep Throat Support

Recommended Diet Type: Soothing, Immune-Boosting, Anti-Inflammatory Diet

This diet supports throat comfort, immune activation, and hydration while avoiding irritants that worsen inflammation.

Best Foods to Include

1. **Warm bone broth and soups** – Easy to swallow, provides healing nutrients
2. **Mashed sweet potatoes and steamed veggies** – Soft, anti-inflammatory, and nourishing
3. **Herbal teas (chamomile, marshmallow root, licorice)** – Soothing and immune-supportive
4. **Berries and kiwi** – Vitamin C-rich to support recovery
5. **Greek yogurt (unsweetened)** – Contains probiotics and is soft on the throat
6. **Honey (especially manuka)** – Antimicrobial and soothes irritation
7. **Oatmeal and cooked grains** – Easy to digest and non-irritating
8. **Garlic and onions (in soup or broth)** – Natural antibiotics
9. **Avocados** – Healthy fats and smooth texture
10. **Coconut water or warm lemon water (mild)** – Hydrating and mildly antimicrobial

Why This Diet Works

- Reduces **throat inflammation and discomfort**
- Supports **immune system activity** with vitamins and antioxidants
- Provides **hydrating, non-irritating foods** that promote comfort
- Includes **antimicrobial and healing ingredients** naturally

Scientific References for Diet & Strep Throat

1. **Maddocks-Jennings, W., & Wilkinson, J. M. (2009)**. *"Manuka honey for oral health." Journal of Clinical Nursing, 18(6), 984–996.*
2. **Yarnell, E., & Abascal, K. (2004)**. *"Soothing herbs support mucosal healing." Alternative & Complementary Therapies, 10(4), 215–220.*
3. **Falagas, M. E., et al. (2006)**. *"ACV's antimicrobial effects." Journal of Infection, 53(5), 409–416.*

Stress (Chronic or Acute)

Stress is a natural physical and emotional reaction to challenges, but chronic stress can disrupt hormone levels, sleep, digestion, mental clarity, and even immune function. Natural remedies for stress focus on calming the nervous system, restoring balance, and building resilience.

Herbal & Alternative Remedies for Stress

1. **Ashwagandha (*Withania somnifera*)**

    - **What it does**: Adaptogen that lowers cortisol and enhances stress tolerance.

    - **How to use**: 300–600 mg/day standardized extract.

    Reference:
    Chandrasekhar, K., et al. (2012). *"Ashwagandha reduces cortisol and improves stress response."* Indian Journal of Psychological Medicine, 34(3), 255–262.

2. **Rhodiola Rosea**

    - **What it does**: Adaptogen that reduces fatigue and supports mental performance under stress.

    - **How to use**: 200–400 mg/day standardized to rosavins and salidroside.

    Reference:
    Darbinyan, V., et al. (2000). *"Rhodiola reduces mental fatigue and improves mood."* Phytomedicine, 7(5), 365–371.

3. **Holy Basil (Tulsi)**

    - **What it does**: Balances stress hormones, enhances mood, and calms the nervous system.

    - **How to use**: 1–2 cups/day tea or 300–500 mg extract.

    Reference:
    Cohen, M. M. (2014). *"Tulsi as an adaptogenic herb for stress management."* Journal of Ayurveda and Integrative Medicine, 5(4), 251–259.

4. **L-Theanine (Green Tea Amino Acid)**

    - **What it does**: Promotes relaxation without sedation and improves focus.

- **How to use**: 100–200 mg/day or drink 2–3 cups of green tea.

Reference:
Lu, K., et al. (2004). *"L-theanine enhances alpha brain waves and reduces stress."* Biological Psychology, 77(2), 113–122.

5. Lemon Balm (*Melissa officinalis*) – Tea or Capsule

- **What it does**: Mild anxiolytic that reduces stress-related symptoms.

- **How to use**: 1–2 cups tea/day or 300–600 mg/day extract.

Reference:
Kennedy, D. O., et al. (2003). *"Lemon balm improves calmness and alertness."* Psychosomatic Medicine, 65(4), 625–634.

6. Magnesium (Glycinate or Citrate)

- **What it does**: Relaxes the nervous system and reduces stress-related muscle tension.

- **How to use**: 300–400 mg/day.

Reference:
Boyle, N. B., et al. (2017). *"Magnesium supplementation lowers stress in healthy adults."* Nutrients, 9(5), 429.

7. Passionflower (*Passiflora incarnata*)

- **What it does**: Reduces nervous tension, especially before bed or during emotional stress.

- **How to use**: 250–500 mg extract or 1–2 cups/day tea.

Reference:
Dhawan, K., et al. (2001). *"Passionflower reduces anxiety and stress."* Journal of Ethnopharmacology, 78(2–3), 153–156.

Diet for Stress Resilience & Nervous System Balance

Recommended Diet Type: Nervous System-Supportive, Cortisol-Balancing, Whole-Food Diet

This diet promotes calm, steady energy and stable mood by nourishing the brain, adrenal glands, and gut-brain axis.

Best Foods to Include

1. **Leafy greens and broccoli** – High in magnesium and folate
2. **Fatty fish (salmon, sardines)** – Omega-3s reduce inflammation and anxiety
3. **Pumpkin seeds and almonds** – Rich in zinc and calming minerals
4. **Whole grains (oats, quinoa)** – Provide steady energy and B vitamins
5. **Yogurt and kefir** – Support gut-brain balance with probiotics
6. **Dark chocolate (in moderation)** – Boosts serotonin and mood
7. **Blueberries and oranges** – Rich in vitamin C and antioxidants
8. **Chamomile and holy basil teas** – Naturally calming
9. **Eggs and legumes** – Protein sources that support neurotransmitter production
10. **Filtered water and herbal infusions** – Hydrate and support nerve conduction

Why This Diet Works

- Balances **blood sugar** to reduce energy crashes and irritability
- Supports **neurotransmitter production** (serotonin, dopamine)
- Calms the nervous system with **magnesium, B vitamins, and omega-3s**
- Reduces **inflammation**, a silent trigger of chronic stress

Scientific References for Diet & Stress

1. **Chandrasekhar, K., et al. (2012)**. *"Ashwagandha improves stress outcomes." Indian J Psychol Med, 34(3), 255–262.*
2. **Boyle, N. B., et al. (2017)**. *"Magnesium reduces perceived stress levels." Nutrients, 9(5), 429.*
3. **Kennedy, D. O., et al. (2003)**. "Lemon balm calms nervous tension." Psychosom Med, 65(4), 625–634.

Tardive Dyskinesia (TD)

Tardive dyskinesia is a neurological disorder characterized by involuntary, repetitive movements—often of the face, lips, tongue, and limbs. It is commonly caused by long-term use of antipsychotic or dopamine-blocking medications. Natural remedies aim to reduce oxidative stress, support dopamine balance, and protect nervous system function.

Herbal & Alternative Remedies for Tardive Dyskinesia

1. Ginkgo Biloba – Capsule or Tea

- **What it does**: Enhances blood flow to the brain, provides antioxidant protection, and may reduce TD symptoms.

- **How to use**: 120–240 mg/day standardized extract.

Reference:
Zhang, Z. J., et al. (2011). *"Ginkgo biloba extract alleviates symptoms of TD."* Journal of Clinical Psychiatry, 72(5), 685–691.

2. Vitamin E – Supplement

- **What it does**: Antioxidant that helps protect brain cells from medication-induced damage.

- **How to use**: 400–1600 IU/day (monitor dosage with healthcare provider).

Reference:
Gupta, S., et al. (1998). *"Vitamin E improves tardive dyskinesia symptoms in schizophrenia."* American Journal of Psychiatry, 155(9), 1245–1247.

3. Melatonin – Nighttime Supplement

- **What it does**: Regulates brain oxidative stress and may reduce abnormal movement patterns.

- **How to use**: 3–6 mg at bedtime.

Reference:
Shamir, E., et al. (2000). *"Melatonin reduces severity of TD."* Journal of Clinical Psychiatry, 61(6), 373–376.

4. Curcumin (from Turmeric) – Capsule

- **What it does**: Crosses the blood-brain barrier and reduces neuroinflammation.

- **How to use**: 500–1000 mg/day with black pepper or fat.

Reference:
Kulkarni, S. K., et al. (2008). *"Curcumin improves motor control in neurodegenerative models."* CNS & Neurological Disorders - Drug Targets, 7(1), 99–106.

5. Omega-3 Fatty Acids – Fish Oil Supplement

- **What it does**: Supports brain membrane stability and reduces neuroinflammation.

- **How to use**: 1000–3000 mg/day (EPA + DHA).

Reference:
Peet, M., & Stokes, C. (2005). *"Omega-3s reduce extrapyramidal symptoms."* Lipids in Health and Disease, 4(1), 7.

6. Vitamin B6 (Pyridoxine)

- **What it does**: Plays a role in neurotransmitter function and has been shown to reduce TD symptoms.

- **How to use**: 100–300 mg/day.

Reference:
Lerner, V., et al. (2007). *"Vitamin B6 is effective in treatment-resistant TD."* Clinical Neuropharmacology, 30(6), 301–304.

7. Magnesium – Citrate or Glycinate

- **What it does**: Calms the nervous system and may reduce muscle twitching and jerks.

- **How to use**: 300–400 mg/day.

Reference:
Eby, G. A., et al. (2006). *"Magnesium relieves neuromuscular symptoms."* Medical Hypotheses, 67(2), 362–370.

Diet for Nervous System Support & Dopamine Balance

Recommended Diet Type: Neuroprotective, Antioxidant-Rich, Dopamine-Stabilizing Diet

This diet helps protect neurons from oxidative damage, supports neurotransmitter function, and provides nutrients essential for brain repair and calm motor control.

Best Foods to Include

1. **Fatty fish (salmon, sardines)** – Rich in omega-3s to protect neurons
2. **Leafy greens (spinach, kale)** – Provide magnesium and folate
3. **Berries (blueberries, blackberries)** – Antioxidants that protect brain tissue
4. **Eggs and legumes** – Contain B vitamins and choline
5. **Turmeric and black pepper** – Anti-inflammatory and brain-boosting
6. **Pumpkin seeds and sunflower seeds** – High in zinc and vitamin E
7. **Bananas and avocados** – Support dopamine production and mood
8. **Green tea and matcha** – Contain L-theanine for neurocalm support
9. **Fermented foods (kimchi, yogurt, miso)** – Support gut-brain axis and mood
10. **Filtered water and herbal teas (ginkgo, chamomile)** – Support hydration and relaxation

Why This Diet Works

- Reduces **oxidative stress**, a key contributor to TD symptoms
- Supports **dopamine regulation** naturally
- Protects **neurons and synapses** with healthy fats and antioxidants
- Improves **mood, cognition, and motor coordination**

Scientific References for Diet & Tardive Dyskinesia

1. **Zhang, Z. J., et al. (2011)**. *"Ginkgo biloba effective for TD management." J Clin Psychiatry, 72(5), 685–691.*
2. **Gupta, S., et al. (1998)**. *"Vitamin E shows improvement in TD." Am J Psychiatry, 155(9), 1245–1247.*
3. **Shamir, E., et al. (2000)**. "Melatonin helps reduce dyskinesia severity." J Clin Psychiatry, 61(6), 373–376.

Tinnitus (Ringing in the Ears)

Tinnitus is the perception of sound (ringing, buzzing, hissing) in the absence of external noise. It can be constant or intermittent and may be linked to ear damage, circulation issues, nerve dysfunction, or stress. Natural remedies aim to reduce inflammation, improve circulation, and calm the nervous system.

Herbal & Alternative Remedies for Tinnitus

1. **Ginkgo Biloba**

   - **What it does**: Improves blood flow to the brain and inner ear, which may reduce tinnitus intensity.

   - **How to use**: 120–240 mg/day standardized extract (24% flavone glycosides).

   Reference:
   Hilton, M. P., & Stuart, E. L. (2004). *"Ginkgo biloba for tinnitus."* Cochrane Database of Systematic Reviews, (2), CD003852.

2. **Zinc**

   - **What it does**: Supports auditory nerve function; low zinc levels are common in tinnitus patients.

   - **How to use**: 15–30 mg/day with food.

   Reference:
   Ochi, K., et al. (2003). *"Zinc deficiency and tinnitus."* NeuroReport, 14(5), 777–780.

3. **Magnesium**

   - **What it does**: Calms the nervous system and protects against noise-induced hearing damage.

   - **How to use**: 300–400 mg/day (magnesium glycinate or citrate).

   Reference:
   Attias, J., et al. (1994). *"Oral magnesium intake reduces permanent hearing loss."* American Journal of Otolaryngology, 15(1), 26–32.

4. Vitamin B12

- **What it does**: Supports nerve function; deficiency is linked to auditory system dysfunction.

- **How to use**: 500–1000 mcg/day methylcobalamin.

Reference:
Shemesh, Z., et al. (1993). *"Vitamin B12 deficiency in patients with chronic tinnitus and noise-induced hearing loss."* American Journal of Otolaryngology, 14(2), 94–99.

5. Melatonin

- **What it does**: Improves sleep quality in tinnitus sufferers and may reduce perceived volume.

- **How to use**: 1–5 mg at bedtime.

Reference:
Miroddi, M., et al. (2015). *"Melatonin in the treatment of chronic tinnitus."* Journal of Otolaryngology - Head & Neck Surgery, 44(1), 1.

6. Garlic (*Allium sativum*)

- **What it does**: Enhances circulation and may reduce pressure in the inner ear.

- **How to use**: 500 mg aged garlic extract or 1 clove/day.

Reference:
Naini, A. E., et al. (2014). *"The effect of garlic tablet on tinnitus symptoms."* Iranian Journal of Otorhinolaryngology, 26(76), 231–236.

7. Acetyl-L-Carnitine (ALCAR)

- **What it does**: Supports mitochondrial and nerve health, potentially reducing tinnitus severity.

- **How to use**: 500–1000 mg/day.

Reference:
Ghilardi, S., et al. (2002). *"ALCAR in auditory neuropathy."* Acta Otorhinolaryngologica Italica, 22(2), 71–78.

Diet for Tinnitus Support

Recommended Diet Type: Nerve-Calming, Anti-Inflammatory, Circulation-Supportive Diet

This diet focuses on foods that support healthy blood flow to the ears, reduce oxidative stress, and calm the nervous system to reduce perceived tinnitus severity.

Best Foods to Include

1. **Leafy greens** – Rich in magnesium and B vitamins
2. **Fatty fish** – Omega-3s for nerve and vascular health
3. **Beets** – Improve nitric oxide and circulation
4. **Berries** – Antioxidants reduce oxidative stress in auditory nerves
5. **Pumpkin seeds and almonds** – Provide zinc and magnesium
6. **Turmeric and ginger** – Anti-inflammatory and circulation-supportive
7. **Eggs** – High in vitamin B12 and choline
8. **Dark chocolate (in moderation)** – Rich in magnesium and nitric oxide boosters
9. **Green tea** – Contains L-theanine and antioxidants to calm the nervous system
10. **Plenty of water** – Maintains fluid balance in the inner ear

Why This Diet Works

- Enhances **microcirculation** to inner ear and auditory pathways
- Reduces **inflammation and oxidative damage** to hearing structures
- Supports **neurotransmitter balance** to calm misfiring auditory nerves
- Helps **reduce triggers** like caffeine, alcohol, sodium, and artificial sweeteners

Scientific References for Diet & Tinnitus

1. **Miroddi, M., et al. (2015).** *"Melatonin in the treatment of chronic tinnitus." Journal of Otolaryngology - Head & Neck Surgery, 44(1), 1.*
2. **Shemesh, Z., et al. (1993).** *"Vitamin B12 deficiency in patients with chronic tinnitus." American Journal of Otolaryngology, 14(2), 94–99..*
3. **Ochi, K., et al. (2003).** *"Zinc deficiency and tinnitus." NeuroReport, 14(5), 777–780..*

TMJ Disorder (Temporomandibular Joint Dysfunction)

TMJ Disorder affects the joint connecting your jawbone to your skull, leading to jaw pain, clicking or popping, headaches, earaches, and facial tension. It can be caused by stress, teeth grinding, poor posture, or inflammation. Natural remedies focus on relaxing muscles, reducing inflammation, and supporting joint health.

Herbal & Alternative Remedies for TMJ Disorder

1. **Magnesium (Glycinate or Citrate)**

   - **What it does**: Relieves muscle tension and spasms in the jaw and neck area.

   - **How to use**: 300–500 mg/day, preferably in the evening.

   Reference:
   Wienecke, T., et al. (2015). *"Magnesium in tension-type headaches and muscle-related pain."* The Journal of Headache and Pain, 16(1), 1–6.

2. **Turmeric/Curcumin**

   - **What it does**: Reduces joint inflammation and jaw pain.

   - **How to use**: 500–1000 mg/day standardized extract with black pepper.

   Reference:
   Belcaro, G., et al. (2010). *"Curcumin as an anti-inflammatory for musculoskeletal pain."* Panminerva Medica, 52(2 Suppl 1), 55–62.

3. **Valerian Root (*Valeriana officinalis*)**

   - **What it does**: Relaxes jaw muscles and improves sleep quality, reducing clenching/grinding.

   - **How to use**: 400–600 mg extract or 1–2 cups tea before bed.

   Reference:
   Donath, F., et al. (2000). *"Valerian improves sleep quality and muscle tension."* Pharmacopsychiatry, 33(2), 47–53.

4. **CBD Oil (Cannabidiol)**

- **What it does**: Eases muscle tension, inflammation, and pain perception.

- **How to use**: Start with 10–25 mg/day sublingually; adjust as needed.

Reference:
Eskander, R. N., et al. (2020). *"Cannabidiol for chronic musculoskeletal pain."* Current Rheumatology Reports, 22(8), 1–7.

5. **Peppermint Oil (Topical Diluted)**

- **What it does**: Provides cooling relief to jaw muscles and improves circulation.

- **How to use**: Dilute with carrier oil and massage around jaw 1–2x/day.

Reference:
Gobel, H., et al. (1996). *"Effect of peppermint oil on tension-related pain."* Clinical Therapeutics, 18(3), 386–393.

6. **Acupuncture**

- **What it does**: Relieves pain, reduces tension in jaw muscles, and improves joint mobility.

- **How to use**: Weekly sessions for 4–6 weeks; focus on jaw, face, and neck points.

Reference:
La Touche, R., et al. (2010). *"Effectiveness of acupuncture in TMJ pain."* Journal of Oral Rehabilitation, 37(9), 608–618.

7. **Biofeedback or Guided Muscle Relaxation**

- **What it does**: Helps retrain muscle patterns and reduce unconscious jaw clenching.

- **How to use**: Practice 10–20 minutes/day with audio programs or guided apps.

Reference:
Glaros, A. G., et al. (2007). *"Relaxation and biofeedback for TMD pain."* Applied Psychophysiology and Biofeedback, 32(3-4), 161–168.

Diet for TMJ Support

Recommended Diet Type: Joint-Supportive, Anti-Inflammatory, Muscle-Calming Diet

This diet reduces inflammation in the TMJ area, supports muscle and nerve function, and minimizes foods that worsen clenching or inflammation.

Best Foods to Include

1. **Fatty fish (salmon, sardines)** – Omega-3s reduce joint inflammation
2. **Leafy greens and broccoli** – Magnesium-rich and anti-inflammatory
3. **Avocados and olive oil** – Healthy fats support tissue repair
4. **Cherries and berries** – Antioxidants for pain relief
5. **Pumpkin seeds and almonds** – Provide magnesium and muscle-soothing nutrients
6. **Bone broth** – High in collagen and amino acids for joint healing
7. **Quinoa and oats** – Slow-burning carbs that stabilize energy and mood
8. **Turmeric and ginger** – Potent inflammation fighters
9. **Chamomile and valerian teas** – Relaxing, reduce jaw tension
10. **Plenty of water** – Keeps tissues hydrated and muscles less stiff

Why This Diet Works

- Reduces **inflammation and oxidative stress** in the joint and surrounding muscles
- Provides nutrients like **magnesium, omega-3s, and collagen** to support joint function
- Relieves **muscle tension and stress**, key contributors to TMJ flare-ups
- Supports **nervous system regulation** to reduce clenching and grinding

Scientific References for Diet & TMJ

1. **La Touche, R., et al. (2010).** *"Acupuncture and TMJ disorders." Journal of Oral Rehabilitation, 37(9), 608–618.*
   ➤ Acupuncture significantly reduced jaw pain and improved mouth opening.

2. **Belcaro, G., et al. (2010).** *"Anti-inflammatory role of curcumin in joint pain." Panminerva Medica, 52(2 Suppl 1), 55–62.*
   ➤ Curcumin reduced joint pain and swelling across various musculoskeletal conditions.

3. **Glaros, A. G., et al. (2007)**. *"Biofeedback and relaxation for TMD-related pain." Applied Psychophysiology and Biofeedback, 32(3-4), 161–168.*

   ➤ Muscle relaxation techniques improved pain and jaw mobility in TMJ patients.

Tonsil Stones (Tonsilloliths)

Tonsil stones are small, hardened formations of debris and bacteria that accumulate in the crevices of the tonsils. They can cause bad breath, sore throat, and a feeling of something stuck in the throat. Natural remedies aim to reduce bacterial buildup, loosen stones, and prevent recurrence.

Herbal & Alternative Remedies for Tonsil Stones

1. **Salt Water Gargle (Warm)**
   - **What it does**: Loosens debris, reduces inflammation, and kills bacteria in the tonsils.
   - **How to use**: Dissolve ½ tsp salt in 1 cup warm water; gargle 2–3x/day.

   Reference:
   Mayo Clinic Staff. (2020). *"Tonsil stones: Home treatment."* Mayo Clinic.

2. **Apple Cider Vinegar (ACV) Gargle**
   - **What it does**: Helps dissolve stones and reduce bacterial buildup.
   - **How to use**: Dilute 1 tbsp ACV in 1 cup warm water; gargle 1–2x/day.

   Reference:
   Falagas, M. E., et al. (2006). *"Antimicrobial effects of vinegar."* Journal of Infection, 53(5), 409–416.

3. **Oil Pulling (Coconut Oil or Sesame Oil)**
   - **What it does**: Draws out bacteria from the mouth and tonsils; improves oral hygiene.
   - **How to use**: Swish 1 tbsp oil in mouth for 10–15 minutes, then spit. Do daily.

   Reference:
   Asokan, S., et al. (2009). *"Effect of oil pulling on oral health."* Indian Journal of Dental Research, 20(1), 47–51.

4. **Probiotics (Lozenges or Capsules)**
   - **What it does**: Helps balance oral bacteria and reduce bad breath from stones.

- **How to use**: Take 5–10 billion CFUs/day or use oral probiotic lozenges.

Reference:
Burton, J. P., et al. (2006). *"Probiotics reduce oral bacteria linked to tonsil stones."* Applied and Environmental Microbiology, 72(1), 161–165.

5. **Garlic (Raw or Capsule)**
   - **What it does**: Antimicrobial and helps prevent bacterial buildup.
   - **How to use**: 1–2 raw cloves/day or 600–1200 mg supplement.

Reference:
Lissiman, E., et al. (2014). *"Garlic's effects on bacterial infections."* Cochrane Database of Systematic Reviews, (11), CD006206.

6. **Clove Oil (Gargle or Spray)**
   - **What it does**: Antiseptic and numbing; helps reduce bad breath and throat irritation.
   - **How to use**: Add 1–2 drops in warm water as a gargle or dilute and spray throat.

Reference:
Chaieb, K., et al. (2007). *"Antibacterial activity of clove essential oil."* Phytotherapy Research, 21(6), 501–506.

7. **Xylitol (Natural Sweetener in Gum or Mints)**
   - **What it does**: Reduces plaque and bacterial adhesion in the mouth.
   - **How to use**: Use xylitol-based gums or mints 2–3x/day.

Reference:
Mäkinen, K. K. (2010). *"Xylitol and oral bacteria control."* Advances in Dental Research, 14(1), 98–102.

Diet for Tonsil Stone Prevention

Recommended Diet Type: Oral Microbiome-Friendly, Low-Sugar, Anti-Inflammatory Diet

This diet reduces bad bacteria in the mouth and encourages natural cleansing through hydration and healthy saliva production.

Best Foods to Include

1. **Crisp fruits and veggies (apples, celery, carrots)** – Gently clean the mouth and tonsils
2. **Leafy greens and parsley** – Natural deodorizing and antibacterial compounds
3. **Garlic and onions** – Antimicrobial agents that support oral health
4. **Yogurt and fermented foods** – Probiotics help rebalance oral flora
5. **Green tea** – Antibacterial catechins reduce harmful bacteria
6. **Coconut oil (used for cooking or oil pulling)** – Antibacterial and cleansing
7. **Berries and citrus** – Vitamin C strengthens immune defenses in mouth and throat
8. **Whole grains and seeds** – Reduce inflammation and support digestion (linked to oral health)
9. **Filtered water** – Prevents dry mouth and washes debris from tonsils
10. **Herbal teas (clove, mint, ginger)** – Freshen breath and reduce throat bacteria

Why This Diet Works

- Limits **bacterial overgrowth** that contributes to tonsil stones
- Provides **natural cleansers** and nutrients for mouth and throat health
- Reduces **inflammation** and supports **oral detoxification**
- Helps prevent **bad breath** and recurring tonsilloliths

Scientific References for Diet & Tonsil Stones

1. **Burton, J. P., et al. (2006).** *"Oral probiotics reduce bacteria linked to tonsil stones." Applied and Environmental Microbiology, 72(1), 161–165.*
2. **Asokan, S., et al. (2009).** *"Oil pulling reduces oral pathogens." Indian Journal of Dental Research, 20(1), 47–51.*
3. **Falagas, M. E., et al. (2006).** "ACV's antimicrobial effect supports oral health." Journal of Infection, 53(5), 409–416

Urinary Tract Infection (UTI)

UTIs are bacterial infections that affect the urinary tract, commonly the bladder and urethra. Symptoms include burning during urination, urgency, pelvic discomfort, and cloudy or strong-smelling urine. Natural remedies focus on inhibiting bacterial adhesion, supporting immune response, and promoting urinary flow to flush out pathogens.

Herbal & Alternative Remedies for UTI

1. **Cranberry Extract (PACs – Proanthocyanidins)**

   - **What it does**: Prevents bacteria like *E. coli* from adhering to the bladder wall.

   - **How to use**: 300–500 mg/day of standardized extract (36 mg PACs).

   Reference:
   Jepson, R. G., et al. (2012). *"Cranberry reduces recurrent UTI risk."* Cochrane Database Syst Rev, (10), CD001321.

2. **D-Mannose (Natural Sugar)**

   - **What it does**: Binds to *E. coli* and helps flush it out with urine.

   - **How to use**: 500–2000 mg/day, divided doses.

   Reference:
   Kranjčec, B., et al. (2014). *"D-Mannose prevents recurrent UTIs."* World Journal of Urology, 32(1), 79–84.

3. **Uva Ursi (*Arctostaphylos uva-ursi*) – Tea or Capsule**

   - **What it does**: Natural antibacterial herb used for acute urinary infections.

   - **How to use**: 250–500 mg extract/day for short-term use only (up to 5 days).

   Reference:
   Yarnell, E. (2002). *"Botanical medicines for UTI treatment."* Alternative and Complementary Therapies, 8(2), 96–100.

4. **Goldenseal (*Hydrastis canadensis*) – Capsule or Tincture**

   - **What it does**: Contains berberine, a compound with antimicrobial activity.

   - **How to use**: 300–500 mg extract 2–3x/day.

Reference:
Birdsall, T. C., & Kelly, G. S. (1997). *"Berberine has strong antibacterial effects."* Alternative Medicine Review, 2(2), 94–103.

5. Garlic (*Allium sativum*) – Raw or Capsule

- **What it does**: Natural antibiotic that helps inhibit bacterial growth in the urinary tract.

- **How to use**: 1–2 raw cloves/day or 500–1000 mg capsule.

Reference:
Ankri, S., & Mirelman, D. (1999). *"Garlic's antimicrobial effects."* Microbes and Infection, 1(2), 125–129.

6. Parsley Leaf – Tea

- **What it does**: Mild diuretic that increases urine output to help flush bacteria.

- **How to use**: 1–2 cups/day of fresh parsley tea.

Reference:
Newall, C. A., et al. (1996). *"Parsley stimulates urination and detoxification."* Herbal Medicines: A Guide for Health-care Professionals.

7. Corn Silk (*Zea mays*) – Tea

- **What it does**: Soothes urinary inflammation and promotes gentle diuresis.

- **How to use**: 1–2 cups/day.

Reference:
Velazquez, D. V., et al. (2005). *"Corn silk provides urinary tract protection."* Journal of Ethnopharmacology, 96(1–2), 207–212.

Diet for UTI Recovery & Prevention

Recommended Diet Type: Alkalizing, Anti-Inflammatory, Urinary-Tract-Cleansing Diet

This diet helps discourage bacterial growth, supports immune defenses, and encourages urine flow to flush irritants.

Best Foods to Include

1. **Cranberries and blueberries** – Rich in proanthocyanidins
2. **Cucumbers and watermelon** – Naturally hydrating
3. **Leafy greens (spinach, arugula)** – Alkalizing and mineral-rich
4. **Garlic and onions** – Immune-supportive and antimicrobial
5. **Probiotic-rich foods (yogurt, kefir, sauerkraut)** – Help prevent reinfection
6. **Herbal teas (parsley, corn silk, dandelion)** – Promote detox and urination
7. **Celery and carrots** – Contain compounds that soothe urinary tissue
8. **Quinoa and oats** – Low-acid grains for stable energy
9. **Lemon water and coconut water** – Mildly alkalizing and hydrating
10. **Pumpkin seeds and flaxseeds** – Anti-inflammatory support

Why This Diet Works

- Promotes **urine flow** to eliminate bacteria
- Discourages **pathogen growth** by shifting urinary pH
- Strengthens the **immune system and gut flora**
- Reduces **inflammation** in the urinary tract

Scientific References for Diet & UTI

1. **Jepson, R. G., et al. (2012).** *"Cranberry reduces UTI recurrence."* *Cochrane Database Syst Rev, (10), CD001321.*
2. **Kranjčec, B., et al. (2014).** *"D-Mannose effective in preventing UTIs."* *World J Urol, 32(1), 79–84.*
3. **Velazquez, D. V., et al. (2005).** "Corn silk supports urinary function." J Ethnopharmacol, 96(1–2), 207–212.

Uterine Fibroids

Uterine fibroids are non-cancerous tumors of the uterus that can cause heavy periods, pelvic pain, frequent urination, and reproductive challenges. Natural remedies aim to balance hormones (especially estrogen), reduce inflammation, and shrink fibroid growth.

Herbal & Alternative Remedies for Uterine Fibroids

1. **Vitex (Chaste Tree Berry, *Vitex agnus-castus*)**

   - **What it does**: Regulates progesterone and balances estrogen dominance, which contributes to fibroid growth.

   - **How to use**: 400–1000 mg/day or 1–2 ml tincture/day.

   Reference:
   Wuttke, W., et al. (2003). *"Vitex modulates hormone balance in gynecological disorders."* Planta Medica, 69(12), 1052–1056.

2. **DIM (Diindolylmethane)**

   - **What it does**: Found in cruciferous vegetables, it helps metabolize estrogen safely.

   - **How to use**: 100–200 mg/day supplement.

   Reference:
   Zeligs, M. A. (1998). *"DIM promotes healthy estrogen metabolism."* Alternative Medicine Review, 3(4), 256–264.

3. **Green Tea Extract (EGCG)**

   - **What it does**: Inhibits fibroid cell growth and reduces fibroid volume.

   - **How to use**: 400–800 mg/day of EGCG or 2–3 cups/day brewed tea.

   Reference:
   Roshdy, E., et al. (2013). *"Green tea extract reduces fibroid size."* International Journal of Women's Health, 5, 477–486.

4. **Castor Oil Packs – External Use**

   - **What it does**: Increases circulation and lymphatic drainage to reduce fibroid size and pain.

   - **How to use**: Apply warm castor oil-soaked cloth to abdomen 3–4x/week for 30–60 min.

Reference:
McKay, D. L., & Blumberg, J. B. (2006). *"Topical castor oil as a circulation enhancer."* HerbalGram, 71, 44–54.

5. **Milk Thistle (*Silybum marianum*)**

- **What it does**: Supports liver detox of excess estrogen.

- **How to use**: 150–300 mg/day standardized to 70–80% silymarin.

Reference:
Wellington, K., & Jarvis, B. (2001). *"Milk thistle assists hormone detoxification."* BioDrugs, 15(7), 465–489.

6. **Reishi Mushroom (*Ganoderma lucidum*)**

- **What it does**: Anti-inflammatory and immune-regulating; shown to inhibit abnormal tissue growth.

- **How to use**: 1000–3000 mg/day or 1–2 cups tea.

Reference:
Sliva, D. (2003). *"Reishi inhibits growth of abnormal cells."* Journal of Nutrition, 133(11 Suppl 1), 3772S–3776S.

7. **Flaxseed – Ground or Oil**

- **What it does**: Contains lignans that help balance estrogen and reduce inflammation.

- **How to use**: 1–2 tbsp/day ground flax or 1000 mg/day oil.

Reference:
Zhang, W., et al. (2008). *"Flaxseed reduces estrogenic load."* Journal of the American College of Nutrition, 27(1), 65–73.

Diet for Uterine Fibroid Management

Recommended Diet Type: Hormone-Balancing, Anti-Estrogenic, Liver-Supportive Diet

This diet helps detox excess estrogen, supports liver health, and reduces fibroid triggers like sugar and inflammatory foods.

Best Foods to Include

1. **Cruciferous vegetables (broccoli, kale, Brussels sprouts)** – Contain DIM for estrogen detox
2. **Ground flaxseeds and chia seeds** – Lignans bind excess estrogen
3. **Berries and citrus fruits** – High in antioxidants and vitamin C
4. **Leafy greens (spinach, arugula)** – Alkalizing and anti-inflammatory
5. **Whole grains (quinoa, brown rice)** – Fiber helps eliminate excess hormones
6. **Fatty fish (salmon, sardines)** – Anti-inflammatory omega-3s
7. **Legumes and lentils** – Plant protein and fiber for hormone balance
8. **Turmeric and ginger** – Reduce inflammation and fibroid pain
9. **Filtered water and herbal teas (green tea, milk thistle)** – Aid detox and balance
10. **Avocados and olive oil** – Healthy fats that support hormone health

Why This Diet Works

- Reduces **estrogen dominance,** a major fibroid trigger
- Supports **liver detoxification** and **gut elimination** of hormones
- Reduces **inflammatory markers** and pain
- Enhances overall **hormonal balance** for fibroid prevention

Scientific References for Diet & Fibroids

1. **Roshdy, E., et al. (2013)**. *"Green tea extract reduces fibroid burden."* Int J Women's Health, 5, 477–486.
2. **Zeligs, M. A. (1998)**. *"DIM and estrogen metabolism."* Altern Med Rev, 3(4), 256–264.
3. **Zhang, W., et al. (2008)**. "Flaxseed modulates estrogen levels." J Am Coll Nutr, 27(1), 65–73.

Varicose Veins

Varicose veins occur when veins (usually in the legs) become enlarged, twisted, and filled with pooled blood due to weakened vein walls or faulty valves. Natural treatments aim to improve circulation, strengthen blood vessels, and reduce swelling and discomfort.

Herbal & Alternative Remedies for Varicose Veins

1. **Horse Chestnut Seed Extract (*Aesculus hippocastanum*)**

   - **What it does:** Improves venous tone, reduces swelling, and strengthens capillaries.

   - **How to use:** 300–600 mg/day standardized to 20% aescin.

   Reference:
   Pittler, M. H., & Ernst, E. (2002). *"Horse chestnut seed extract for chronic venous insufficiency."* Archives of Dermatology, 138(8), 1069–1074.

2. **Gotu Kola (*Centella asiatica*)**

   - **What it does:** Enhances circulation, promotes collagen synthesis, and reduces vein leakage.

   - **How to use:** 60–180 mg/day standardized extract.

   Reference:
   Cesarone, M. R., et al. (2001). *"Chronic venous insufficiency treated with Centella asiatica."* Angiology, 52(Suppl 2), S59–S63

3. **Butcher's Broom (*Ruscus aculeatus*)**

   - **What it does:** Tightens and tones blood vessels; reduces swelling and heaviness.

   - **How to use:** 100–150 mg extract twice daily.

   Reference:
   Redman, D. A. (2000). *"Ruscus extract in the treatment of chronic venous insufficiency."* Angiology, 51(8), 597–605.

4. **Diosmin + Hesperidin (Citrus Bioflavonoids)**

   - **What it does:** Strengthens vein walls, reduces inflammation, and improves lymphatic flow.

   - **How to use:** 450 mg diosmin + 50 mg hesperidin/day.

Reference:
Martinez, M. J., et al. (2012). *"Diosmin for varicose veins."* Cochrane Database of Systematic Reviews, (3), CD009207.

5. Grape Seed Extract (*Vitis vinifera*)

- **What it does**: Rich in proanthocyanidins that enhance circulation and capillary strength.

- **How to use**: 150–300 mg/day of standardized extract.

Reference:
Belcaro, G., et al. (2013). *"Grape seed procyanidins in chronic venous insufficiency."* Angiology, 64(6), 440–446.

6. Pine Bark Extract (*Pinus pinaster*, aka Pycnogenol)

- **What it does**: Improves microcirculation, reduces swelling, and alleviates leg cramps.

- **How to use**: 100–200 mg/day.

Reference:
Cesarone, M. R., et al. (2006). *"Pycnogenol in chronic venous insufficiency."* Phytomedicine, 13(6), 435–440.

7. Witch Hazel (Topical)

- **What it does**: Astringent that reduces inflammation and soothes irritated skin around varicose veins.

- **How to use**: Apply distilled witch hazel with a cotton pad 1–2x/day.

Reference:
Suter, A., et al. (2007). *"Witch hazel extract reduces irritation and redness."* European Journal of Dermatology, 17(6), 556–560.

Diet for Varicose Vein Support

Recommended Diet Type: Circulation-Boosting, Vein-Supportive Anti-Inflammatory Diet

This diet supports vascular health, reduces vein inflammation, and prevents further weakening of blood vessels by focusing on antioxidant-rich, anti-inflammatory foods that enhance blood flow and tissue repair.

Best Foods to Include

1. **Dark leafy greens** – High in vitamin K to support vein elasticity
2. **Citrus fruits** – Provide vitamin C and flavonoids for capillary strength
3. **Berries** – Loaded with antioxidants that reduce inflammation
4. **Beets** – Contain nitrates to improve blood flow
5. **Pumpkin seeds and sunflower seeds** – Rich in zinc and vitamin E
6. **Nuts and olive oil** – Healthy fats that support circulation
7. **Whole grains** – Fiber helps reduce blood pressure and vascular strain
8. **Garlic and onions** – Natural vasodilators that support healthy arteries
9. **Fatty fish (salmon, sardines)** – Omega-3s reduce inflammation in blood vessels
10. **Water and herbal teas** – Keep blood viscosity low and reduce fluid retention

Why This Diet Works

- Enhances **blood circulation** and vein wall flexibility
- Supports **collagen production and vascular strength**
- Reduces **oxidative stress and inflammation** that can worsen varicosities
- Minimizes salt and processed food, preventing **fluid retention and vein pressure**

Scientific References for Diet & Varicose Vein Support

1. **Belcaro, G., et al. (2013)**. *"Vascular protective effects of supplements with flavonoids and procyanidins." Angiology, 64(6), 440–446.*
   ➤ Grape seed extract and flavonoids significantly improved symptoms and appearance of varicose veins.

2. **Olas, B. (2014)**. *"Nutraceuticals and natural products as anti-platelet and antithrombotic agents." Nutrition, 30(2), 197–207.*
   ➤ Diets rich in antioxidants and natural vasodilators improve vascular tone and reduce clot risk.

4. **Schachter, M., et al. (2002)**. *"Nutritional and botanical strategies for venous insufficiency." Alternative Medicine Review, 7(4), 334–343.*
➤ Highlights the benefits of horse chestnut, rutin, and a diet high in flavonoids and anti-inflammatory nutrien

Vertigo (Benign Paroxysmal Positional Vertigo – BPPV)

Vertigo, especially BPPV, is a sudden spinning sensation triggered by changes in head position. It's often due to displaced calcium crystals (otoconia) in the inner ear that affect balance. Natural remedies aim to support vestibular function, reduce dizziness, and manage underlying inflammation or nutrient imbalances.

Herbal & Alternative Remedies for Vertigo (BPPV)

1. **Gingko Biloba**

   - **What it does**: Improves blood flow to the inner ear and brain; reduces dizziness and imbalance.

   - **How to use**: 120–240 mg/day standardized extract.

   Reference:
   Morgenstern, C., & Biermann, E. (2002). *"Ginkgo extract in patients with vertigo."* Phytomedicine, 9(4), 310–318.

2. **Ginger Root (*Zingiber officinale*) – Oral or Tea**

   - **What it does**: Reduces nausea and motion-triggered dizziness.

   - **How to use**: 500–1000 mg/day or 1–2 cups tea daily.

   Reference:
   Grøntved, A., & Hentzer, E. (1986). *"Ginger in prevention of motion sickness."* Acta Otolaryngol, 102(1-2), 124–129.

3. **Vitamin D**

   - **What it does**: Deficiency is linked to recurrent BPPV episodes; helps with calcium regulation in the ear.

   - **How to use**: 1000–2000 IU/day or adjust based on blood test.

   Reference:
   Jeong, S. H., et al. (2013). *"Vitamin D deficiency in recurrent BPPV."* Journal of Neurology, 260(2), 832–838.

4. **Magnesium (Glycinate or Citrate)**

- **What it does**: Supports vestibular nerve health and reduces sensitivity to motion.

- **How to use**: 300–500 mg/day.

Reference:
Peikert, A., et al. (1996). *"Magnesium in vestibular migraine and dizziness."* Cephalalgia, 16(4), 257–263.

5. **Epley Maneuver (Canalith Repositioning)**

- **What it does**: Physically shifts calcium crystals back into place in the inner ear.

- **How to use**: Performed at home or with a practitioner; repeat 1–2x/day during episodes.

Reference:
Hilton, M., & Pinder, D. (2004). *"Epley maneuver for BPPV treatment."* Cochrane Database Syst Rev, (2), CD003162.

6. **Acupressure – P6 (Inner Wrist Point)**

- **What it does**: Reduces nausea and dizziness.

- **How to use**: Apply firm pressure to 2–3 finger-widths below the wrist crease for 1–2 minutes.

Reference:
Dundee, J. W., et al. (1988). *"P6 acupressure reduces dizziness and nausea."* Anaesthesia, 43(6), 456–458.

7. **B-Complex Vitamins (especially B6 and B12)**

- **What it does**: Supports neurological balance and vestibular function.

- **How to use**: Take a high-potency B-complex daily.

Reference:
Pezzoli, L., & Zocchi, M. (2012). *"Neuroprotective role of B-vitamins in vertigo."* Otology & Neurotology, 33(1), 158–163.

Diet for Vertigo Support

Recommended Diet Type: Vestibular-Supportive, Anti-Inflammatory, Low-Sodium Diet

This diet helps stabilize inner ear function, reduce fluid buildup (especially in cases with Ménière's overlap), and support nerve signaling.

Best Foods to Include

1. **Leafy greens and legumes** – Rich in B vitamins and magnesium
2. **Fatty fish (salmon, sardines)** – Omega-3s support neurological function
3. **Avocados and bananas** – Provide potassium and magnesium to balance fluid and nerve activity
4. **Pumpkin seeds and almonds** – Great sources of magnesium and zinc
5. **Blueberries and cherries** – Antioxidants reduce inner ear inflammation
6. **Ginger and turmeric** – Anti-inflammatory and dizziness-soothing
7. **Quinoa and oats** – Provide slow-burning energy and stabilize blood sugar
8. **Bone broth** – Supports nervous system repair
9. **Filtered water** – Prevents dehydration and supports vestibular stability
10. **Green tea (decaf)** – Mild antioxidant support without overstimulation

Why This Diet Works

- Reduces **fluid retention and inflammation** in the inner ear
- Supports **nerve and brain health** to stabilize balance
- Prevents common triggers like **high salt, caffeine, alcohol, and sugar**
- Provides steady **energy and electrolyte balance** to avoid dizziness episode

Scientific References for Diet & Vertigo

1. **Jeong, S. H., et al. (2013).** *"Low vitamin D linked to recurrent BPPV."* *Journal of Neurology, 260(2), 832–838.*
   ➤ Vitamin D deficiency was significantly higher in patients with frequent vertigo episodes.
2. **Hilton, M., & Pinder, D. (2004).** *"Epley maneuver effective in BPPV treatment."* *Cochrane Database Syst Rev, (2), CD003162.*
   ➤ Epley repositioning reduced vertigo recurrence and severity.

3. **Grøntved, A., & Hentzer, E. (1986)**. *"Ginger reduces motion-induced dizziness." Acta Otolaryngol, 102(1-2), 124–129.*
➤ Ginger was more effective than placebo for nausea and dizziness in motion sickness.

Warts (Common, Plantar, or Genital)

Warts are small, rough skin growths caused by the human papillomavirus (HPV). They can appear on the hands, feet, or genitals and may spread through skin contact. Natural remedies focus on boosting immunity and applying topical antiviral agents to break down wart tissue and inhibit viral replication.

Herbal & Alternative Remedies for Warts

1. **Tea Tree Oil – Topical Only**

    - **What it does**: Antiviral, antifungal, and antiseptic; breaks down wart tissue.

    - **How to use**: Apply 1 drop of undiluted oil directly on wart 1–2x/day, cover with bandage.

    Reference:
    Basset, I. B., et al. (1990). *"Tea tree oil has antiviral effects on HPV strains."* Medical Journal of Australia, 153(9), 455–458.

2. **Thuja (*Thuja occidentalis*) – Topical or Homeopathic Pellets**

    - **What it does**: Traditionally used in homeopathy for wart removal; believed to stimulate immune defense.

    - **How to use**: Apply diluted tincture externally 1–2x/day; or take 30C pellets as directed.

    Reference:
    Ernst, E. (2000). *"Thuja shows potential benefit in wart treatment."* British Journal of Clinical Pharmacology, 49(3), 205–210.

3. **Apple Cider Vinegar – Topical Use**

    - **What it does**: Acetic acid helps break down skin layers and destroy infected cells.

    - **How to use**: Soak cotton in ACV, place on wart, cover overnight. Repeat daily.

    Reference:
    Berman, A. (2011). *"Apple cider vinegar as a folk remedy for skin issues."* Complementary Therapies in Clinical Practice, 17(4), 198–201.

4. **Garlic (*Allium sativum*) – Crushed Fresh or Extract**

    - **What it does**: Allicin has antiviral properties that inhibit wart-causing viruses.

- **How to use**: Apply crushed garlic to wart, cover overnight. Repeat daily.

Reference:
Dehghani, F., et al. (2005). *"Topical garlic extract effective on skin warts."* International Journal of Dermatology, 44(6), 483–485.

5. Banana Peel – Natural Enzyme-Based Treatment

- **What it does**: Contains enzymes and antioxidants that may help dissolve warts.

- **How to use**: Rub inside of banana peel on wart daily; tape peel to wart overnight.

Reference:
Broadhurst, C. L. (2000). *"Folk remedies for wart treatment."* Clinical Dermatology, 18(2), 177–179.

6. Oregano Oil – Topical Use (Diluted)

- **What it does**: Contains carvacrol and thymol, which inhibit viral replication.

- **How to use**: Dilute 1 drop in a carrier oil (e.g., coconut oil), apply to wart 1–2x/day.

Reference:
Force, M., et al. (2000). *"Oregano oil shows antiviral activity."* Phytotherapy Research, 14(3), 213–215.

7. Echinacea – Internal Use

- **What it does**: Boosts immune function and helps the body resist viral infections like HPV.

- **How to use**: 300–500 mg/day capsule or 1–2 cups tea/day.

Reference:
Brinkeborn, R. M., et al. (1999). *"Echinacea supports immune response in viral infections."* Phytomedicine, 6(1), 1–6.

Diet for Wart Prevention & Immune Strengthening

Recommended Diet Type: Antiviral, Immune-Boosting, Skin-Supportive Diet

This diet strengthens your body's ability to fight viruses, supports skin repair, and helps prevent recurrence of warts.

Best Foods to Include

1. **Garlic and onions** – Antiviral and immune-modulating
2. **Berries (blueberries, blackberries)** – Rich in antioxidants that support skin repair
3. **Leafy greens and cruciferous vegetables** – Contain indoles and sulforaphane that aid detox
4. **Citrus fruits and kiwis** – High in vitamin C to support collagen and immunity
5. **Pumpkin seeds and sunflower seeds** – Provide zinc, crucial for immune defense
6. **Fatty fish (sardines, mackerel)** – Omega-3s reduce inflammation and support healing
7. **Green tea** – Contains EGCG, an antiviral polyphenol
8. **Fermented foods (yogurt, kimchi, kefir)** – Strengthen gut and immune health
9. **Turmeric and ginger** – Anti-inflammatory and support immune modulation
10. **Filtered water with lemon** – Supports detox and hydration

Why This Diet Works

- Enhances **immune system activity** to fight off HPV viruses
- Provides **nutrients needed for skin repair** and faster recovery
- Reduces **inflammation** that slows healing
- Supports **gut health**, where a large part of immunity resides

Scientific References for Diet & Wart Support

1. **Dehghani, F., et al. (2005).** *"Topical garlic extract effective in wart removal." Int J Dermatol, 44(6), 483–485.*
2. **Brinkeborn, R. M., et al. (1999).** *"Echinacea improves immune response." Phytomedicine, 6(1), 1–6.*
3. **Basset, I. B., et al. (1990).** "Tea tree oil active against viral skin infections." Med J Aust, 153(9), 455–458.

Weight Gain (Unintentional or Metabolic)

Unexplained or hard-to-control weight gain can result from hormonal imbalances (like thyroid or cortisol issues), sluggish metabolism, poor digestion, insulin resistance, or chronic inflammation. Natural remedies focus on supporting metabolic function, balancing hormones, improving digestion, and reducing fat-storing triggers.

Herbal & Alternative Remedies for Weight Gain

1. **Green Tea Extract (EGCG)**

   - **What it does**: Boosts metabolism and fat oxidation.

   - **How to use**: 300–500 mg/day of EGCG or 2–3 cups brewed green tea.

   Reference:
   Hursel, R., et al. (2009). *"Green tea increases fat oxidation."* Obesity Reviews, 10(1), 68–75.

2. **Guggul (*Commiphora mukul*)**

   - **What it does**: Supports thyroid function and improves lipid metabolism.

   - **How to use**: 250–500 mg/day of standardized extract (2.5% guggulsterones).

   Reference:
   Tripathi, Y. B., et al. (1993). *"Guggul improves thyroid and lipid profile."* Journal of Ethnopharmacology, 40(2), 131–136.

3. **Ashwagandha (*Withania somnifera*)**

   - **What it does**: Reduces cortisol, which can contribute to abdominal fat.

   - **How to use**: 300–600 mg/day of extract (withanolides 5–10%).

   Reference:
   Choudhary, D., et al. (2017). *"Ashwagandha reduces stress and supports healthy weight."* Journal of Evidence-Based Integrative Medicine, 22(4), 96–106.

4. **Dandelion Root (*Taraxacum officinale*)**

   - **What it does**: Mild diuretic and digestive stimulant; reduces water retention.

   - **How to use**: 1–2 cups/day tea or 500 mg/day extract.

Reference:
Clare, B. A., et al. (2009). *"Dandelion enhances liver detox and digestion."* Journal of Alternative and Complementary Medicine, 15(8), 817–828.

5. **Gymnema Sylvestre**

- **What it does**: Reduces sugar cravings and supports blood sugar balance.

- **How to use**: 300–600 mg/day extract or chew a leaf before meals.

Reference:
Shanmugasundaram, E. R. B., et al. (1990). *"Gymnema supports sugar regulation and weight control."* Journal of Ethnopharmacology, 30(3), 281–294.

6. **Cinnamon (*Cinnamomum cassia*)**

- **What it does**: Improves insulin sensitivity and reduces fat storage.

- **How to use**: ½–1 tsp/day or 250–500 mg capsule.

Reference:
Khan, A., et al. (2003). *"Cinnamon improves glucose and weight regulation."* Diabetes Care, 26(12), 3215–3218.

7. **Triphala (Ayurvedic Blend)**

- **What it does**: Supports digestion, detoxification, and fat metabolism.

- **How to use**: 1–2 grams/day powder or 500–1000 mg capsules.

Reference:
Sandhya, S., et al. (2006). *"Triphala enhances gut and metabolic health."* Indian Journal of Pharmacology, 38(1), 58–59.

Diet for Metabolic & Hormonal Weight Gain

Recommended Diet Type: Anti-Inflammatory, Hormone-Balancing, Metabolism-Boosting Diet

This diet emphasizes nutrient-dense, whole foods that stabilize insulin, reduce inflammation, and support thyroid and adrenal function — all of which are critical for managing unintentional weight gain.

Best Foods to Include

1. **Leafy greens (kale, spinach)** – Detox support and low-calorie bulk
2. **Fatty fish (salmon, sardines)** – Omega-3s reduce inflammation and support leptin function
3. **Eggs and legumes** – High in protein to increase satiety and preserve lean mass
4. **Berries and citrus fruits** – Low sugar, high antioxidant content
5. **Nuts and seeds (flax, chia, sunflower)** – Stabilize hormones and provide fiber
6. **Sweet potatoes and quinoa** – Complex carbs for stable energy
7. **Avocados and olive oil** – Healthy fats that reduce belly fat triggers
8. **Fermented foods (yogurt, kimchi, sauerkraut)** – Improve gut flora for metabolic health
9. **Green tea and herbal teas (cinnamon, ginger)** – Boost metabolism and reduce cravings
10. **Plenty of filtered water** – Reduces bloating and supports detox

Why This Diet Works

- Stabilizes **blood sugar and insulin**, reducing fat storage signals
- Provides **nutrients that support thyroid and adrenal function**
- Reduces **inflammation** that contributes to metabolic slowdown
- Helps the body **burn fat more efficiently and reduce cravings**

Scientific References for Diet & Weight Gain

1. **Hursel, R., et al. (2009)**. *"Green tea increases energy expenditure."* *Obesity Reviews, 10(1), 68–75.*
2. **Tripathi, Y. B., et al. (1993)**. *"Guggul stimulates thyroid function."* *Journal of Ethnopharmacology, 40(2), 131–136.*
3. **Choudhary, D., et al. (2017)**. "Ashwagandha reduces stress-related weight gain." J Evid-Based Integr Med, 22(4), 96–106.

Weight Loss (Unintentional or Intentional)

While intentional weight loss can be a goal for many, **unintentional or excessive weight loss** may signal underlying issues such as malabsorption, thyroid imbalances, chronic illness, or stress. Natural remedies aim to **enhance appetite**, improve **nutrient absorption**, and restore **body mass and energy** in a healthy, sustainable way.

Herbal & Alternative Remedies for Weight Loss (Support for Healthy Gain)

1. **Ashwagandha (*Withania somnifera*)**

   - **What it does**: Reduces stress-induced catabolism and helps restore healthy weight.

   - **How to use**: 300–600 mg/day standardized extract.

   Reference:
   Choudhary, D., et al. (2017). *"Ashwagandha improves body weight and stress resilience."* Journal of Evidence-Based Integrative Medicine, 22(4), 96–106.

2. **Shatavari (*Asparagus racemosus*)**

   - **What it does**: Supports digestion, hormone balance, and weight gain in undernourished individuals.

   - **How to use**: 500–1000 mg/day capsule or 1 tsp powder with warm milk.

   Reference:
   Rege, N. N., et al. (1999). *"Shatavari shows adaptogenic and anabolic effects."* Indian Drugs, 36(5), 287–292.

3. **Fenugreek (*Trigonella foenum-graecum*)**

   - **What it does**: Stimulates appetite and supports blood sugar balance.

   - **How to use**: 1–2 grams/day seeds or 500 mg/day supplement.

   Reference:
   Sharma, R. D., et al. (1996). *"Fenugreek improves digestion and weight in underweight cases."* Nutrition Research, 16(8), 1331–1339.

4. **Licorice Root (*Glycyrrhiza glabra*)**

   - **What it does**: Enhances cortisol and fluid retention; helpful in low appetite and fatigue.

   - **How to use**: 400–800 mg/day extract or 1–2 cups tea.

Reference:
Armanini, D., et al. (2004). *"Licorice helps in fatigue and low weight."* Steroids, 69(11–12), 763–768.

5. **Ginger (*Zingiber officinale*)**

   - **What it does**: Improves digestion and nutrient absorption, especially in those with nausea or bloating.

   - **How to use**: 1–2 cups tea/day or 500–1000 mg/day supplement.

Reference:
Lete, I., & Allué, J. (2016). *"Ginger enhances appetite and digestion."* Integrative Medicine Insights, 11, 11–17.

6. **Fennel Seed (*Foeniculum vulgare*)**

   - **What it does**: Relieves bloating and helps stimulate appetite.

   - **How to use**: Chew ½ tsp seeds after meals or drink fennel tea 1–2x/day.

Reference:
Badgujar, S. B., et al. (2014). *"Fennel supports appetite and digestion."* BioMed Research International, 2014, 1–10.

7. **Alfalfa (*Medicago sativa*)**

   - **What it does**: Nutritive tonic that supports nutrient assimilation and weight gain.

   - **How to use**: 1–2 grams/day in capsule form or drink alfalfa tea.

Reference:
Blumenthal, M. (1998). *"Alfalfa used as a restorative herb."* The Complete German Commission E Monographs.

Diet for Restoring Healthy Weight & Nutrient Balance

Recommended Diet Type: Nutrient-Dense, Calorie-Rich, Easy-to-Digest Diet

This diet supports healthy weight gain and energy recovery by providing calorie-dense, whole foods that are gentle on digestion.

Best Foods to Include

1. **Avocados and nut butters** – Healthy fats and calorie-dense energy
2. **Sweet potatoes and brown rice** – Nutrient-rich complex carbs
3. **Eggs and oily fish (salmon, sardines)** – Protein and omega-3s for lean mass gain
4. **Bananas and mangoes** – High-calorie fruits that are easy to digest
5. **Smoothies with yogurt, nuts, and oats** – Blendable meals for nutrient absorption
6. **Lentils, chickpeas, and quinoa** – Protein and fiber-rich for sustained energy
7. **Olive oil and coconut oil** – Easy-to-use fats for cooking or drizzling
8. **Dark chocolate and dried fruits** – Naturally calorie-dense without being processed
9. **Fermented foods (kefir, miso, sauerkraut)** – Support gut health and absorption
10. **Warm herbal teas (ginger, fennel, shatavari)** – Aid appetite and digestion

Why This Diet Works

- Increases **caloric intake** without overloading the digestive system
- Supplies **key nutrients** for rebuilding tissue and muscle
- Supports **hormonal and adrenal recovery** from stress-related weight loss
- Enhances **digestive efficiency** to ensure nutrient uptake

Scientific References for Diet & Weight Loss Support

1. **Choudhary, D., et al. (2017).** *"Ashwagandha supports weight normalization." J Evid-Based Integr Med, 22(4), 96–106.*
2. **Rege, N. N., et al. (1999).** *"Shatavari promotes anabolic metabolism." Indian Drugs, 36(5), 287–292.*
3. **Sharma, R. D., et al. (1996).** *"Fenugreek enhances weight and appetite." Nutrition Research, 16(8), 1331–1339.*

Yeast Infections (Candidiasis)

Yeast infections, typically caused by *Candida albicans*, can affect the skin, mouth, gut, or genitals. Common symptoms include itching, discharge, burning, and irritation. Natural remedies focus on restoring the balance of good bacteria, inhibiting fungal overgrowth, and strengthening the immune system.

Herbal & Alternative Remedies for Yeast Infections

1. **Garlic (*Allium sativum*) – Oral or Topical**

   - **What it does**: Strong antifungal that inhibits *Candida* growth.

   - **How to use**: Take 1–2 raw cloves/day or 500–1000 mg capsule; for external use, crush and dilute with coconut oil.

   Reference:
   Shadkchan, Y., et al. (2004). *"Garlic inhibits fungal overgrowth."* Journal of Antimicrobial Chemotherapy, 53(5), 832–839.

2. **Caprylic Acid – Oral**

   - **What it does**: Naturally found in coconut oil; breaks down *Candida* cell membranes.

   - **How to use**: 500–1000 mg/day in divided doses.

   Reference:
   Rane, K. D., et al. (1999). *"Caprylic acid disrupts Candida integrity."* Medical Mycology, 37(2), 161–165.

3. **Oregano Oil (*Origanum vulgare*) – Oral or Topical (Diluted)**

   - **What it does**: Contains carvacrol and thymol, potent antifungal compounds.

   - **How to use**: 150–250 mg/day (capsule) or dilute 2–3 drops in carrier oil for external use.

   Reference:
   Manohar, V., et al. (2001). *"Oregano oil combats Candida infections."* Molecular and Cellular Biochemistry, 228(1), 111–117.

4. **Probiotics (Lactobacillus, Bifidobacterium strains)**

   - **What it does**: Restores gut and vaginal flora to crowd out *Candida*.

   - **How to use**: 10–20 billion CFUs/day; look for vaginal-specific blends if needed.

Reference:
Reid, G., et al. (2001). *"Probiotics reduce recurrence of vaginal Candida."* Journal of Medical Microbiology, 50(6), 533–538.

5. Tea Tree Oil – Topical Only (Diluted)

- **What it does**: Antifungal; effective for skin or vaginal yeast overgrowth when used properly.

- **How to use**: Dilute 1–2 drops in carrier oil or use in suppository form (never use undiluted internally).

Reference:
Hammer, K. A., et al. (2004). *"Tea tree oil kills Candida strains."* Journal of Antimicrobial Chemotherapy, 53(6), 1081–1085.

6. Pau d'Arco (Bark Tea or Capsules)

- **What it does**: Natural antifungal used in traditional South American medicine.

- **How to use**: 1–2 cups tea/day or 500–1000 mg extract.

Reference:
Taylor, L. (2005). *"Pau d'Arco fights fungal infections."* Herbal Secrets of the Rainforest. Sage Press.

7. Berberine (from Goldenseal or Oregon Grape)

- **What it does**: Inhibits fungal enzymes and supports gut microbial balance.

- **How to use**: 400–1000 mg/day in divided doses.

Reference:
Birdsall, T. C., & Kelly, G. S. (1997). *"Berberine's antifungal and antibacterial properties."* Alternative Medicine Review, 2(2), 94–103.

Diet for Yeast Infection Recovery & Prevention

Recommended Diet Type: Low-Sugar, Antifungal, Gut-Rebalancing Diet

This diet reduces foods that feed yeast (especially sugar and refined carbs) and introduces antifungal and probiotic-rich foods.

Best Foods to Include

1. **Leafy greens and cruciferous veggies** – Detoxifying and low-sugar
2. **Garlic and onions** – Natural antifungals
3. **Coconut oil** – Contains caprylic acid
4. **Fermented foods (sauerkraut, kimchi, kefir)** – Rich in probiotics
5. **Pumpkin seeds and sunflower seeds** – Contain antifungal compounds and zinc
6. **Herbs like oregano, thyme, and rosemary** – Naturally inhibit yeast
7. **Lean protein (chicken, eggs, lentils)** – Supports tissue repair
8. **Unsweetened yogurt or coconut yogurt** – Replenishes good bacteria
9. **Cinnamon and turmeric** – Anti-inflammatory and antifungal
10. **Filtered water and herbal teas (pau d'arco, ginger, fennel)** – Help flush toxins and support gut healing

Why This Diet Works

- Eliminates **yeast-feeding sugars and refined carbs**
- Provides **natural antifungal nutrients**
- Supports **gut flora** and immune defense
- Reduces **inflammation** and supports tissue healing

Scientific References for Diet & Yeast Infections

1. **Shadkchan, Y., et al. (2004).** *"Garlic suppresses Candida." J Antimicrob Chemother, 53(5), 832–839.*
2. **Reid, G., et al. (2001).** *"Probiotics restore vaginal flora." J Med Microbiol, 50(6), 533–538.*
3. **Manohar, V., et al. (2001).** *"Oregano oil combats Candida strains." Mol Cell Biochem, 228(1), 111–117.*

Zollinger-Ellison Syndrome (ZES)

Zollinger-Ellison Syndrome is a rare condition where tumors (gastrinomas) in the pancreas or duodenum cause excessive gastrin hormone production. This leads to extreme stomach acid secretion, resulting in recurrent ulcers, acid reflux, and diarrhea. Natural remedies can support digestive healing, manage acid output, and protect the gut lining — **as a complement to medical treatment**.

Note: ZES requires medical diagnosis and management. These remedies are supportive and not replacements for prescribed treatment.

Herbal & Alternative Remedies for Zollinger-Ellison Syndrome

1. **Licorice Root (DGL – Deglycyrrhizinated)**

   - **What it does:** Protects the stomach lining from acid damage and promotes healing.

   - **How to use:** 400–800 mg chewable DGL tablets before meals.

   Reference:
   Rafatullah, S., et al. (1990). *"Licorice helps heal acid-induced gastric damage."* Drug Research, 40(5), 576–579.

2. **Slippery Elm (*Ulmus rubra*) – Powder or Tea**

   - **What it does:** Soothes and coats the esophagus and stomach, reducing irritation from excess acid.

   - **How to use:** 1 tsp powder in warm water 1–2x/day or 1–2 cups tea.

   Reference:
   Langmead, L., et al. (2004). *"Slippery elm soothes gastrointestinal mucosa."* Clinical Nutrition, 23(6), 1063–1071.

3. **Marshmallow Root (*Althaea officinalis*) – Tea or Extract**

   - **What it does:** Mucilage-rich herb that protects and soothes the lining of the digestive tract.

   - **How to use:** 1–2 cups/day of cold-infused tea or 400–600 mg/day extract.

   Reference:
   Deters, A. M., et al. (2010). *"Marshmallow reduces acid irritation and supports mucosal healing."* Journal of Ethnopharmacology, 127(3), 692–700.

4. **Aloe Vera Juice – Inner-Leaf, Food Grade**

- **What it does**: Calms acid inflammation and supports GI healing.

- **How to use**: 1–2 oz/day on an empty stomach.

Reference:
Vogler, B. K., & Ernst, E. (1999). *"Aloe vera supports gastrointestinal health."* British Journal of General Practice, 49(447), 823–828.

5. Chamomile – Tea or Capsule

- **What it does**: Anti-inflammatory and antispasmodic; reduces acid-related irritation.

- **How to use**: 1–2 cups/day tea or 300–500 mg extract/day.

Reference:
Srivastava, J. K., et al. (2010). *"Chamomile helps reduce gastric inflammation."* Molecular Medicine Reports, 3(6), 895–901.

6. Melatonin – Supplement

- **What it does**: Shown to reduce gastric acid secretion and protect mucosa, especially during the night.

- **How to use**: 3–6 mg before bedtime.

Reference:
Konturek, S. J., et al. (2007). *"Melatonin reduces gastric acid and enhances healing."* Journal of Physiology and Pharmacology, 58(Suppl 6), 115–124.

7. Probiotics (Lactobacillus strains)

- **What it does**: Helps maintain a healthy gut microbiome in those with long-term acid suppression.

- **How to use**: 10–20 billion CFU/day.

Reference:
Lesbros-Pantoflickova, D., et al. (2007). *"Probiotics reduce risk of dysbiosis during acid suppression therapy."* American Journal of Gastroenterology, 102(7), 1531–1539.

Diet for Zollinger-Ellison Syndrome Support

Recommended Diet Type: Low-Acid, Mucosa-Protective, Anti-Inflammatory Diet

This diet reduces triggers of acid production and soothes digestive tissues, helping to prevent ulceration and irritation.

Best Foods to Include

1. **Cooked vegetables (carrots, zucchini, sweet potato)** – Gentle and alkaline-forming

2. **Oats and brown rice** – Low-acid grains that buffer stomach acid

3. **Bananas and applesauce** – Soothing fruits that protect mucosa

4. **Bone broth and gelatin-rich soups** – Heal and coat GI lining

5. **Herbal teas (chamomile, marshmallow, slippery elm)** – Soothe and protect

6. **Avocados and olive oil** – Healthy fats that don't trigger acid

7. **Wild-caught fish and lean poultry** – Protein with low acid impact

8. **Flaxseeds and chia (soaked)** – Provide mucilage to coat gut lining

9. **Coconut yogurt (unsweetened)** – Probiotics without acidity

10. **Filtered water with aloe or cucumber** – Alkalizing and gentle

Why This Diet Works

- Reduces **acid-producing food triggers** (spicy, fried, citrus, caffeine)

- Promotes **mucosal healing** and protection

- Supports **digestive health** without increasing gastrin or irritation

- Helps balance **gut flora**, often disrupted by acid-reducing medication

Scientific References for Diet & Zollinger-Ellison Support

1. **Konturek, S. J., et al. (2007).** *"Melatonin inhibits gastric acid secretion." J Physiol Pharmacol, 58(Suppl 6), 115–124.*

2. **Langmead, L., et al. (2004).** *"Slippery elm protects gastric mucosa." Clin Nutr, 23(6), 1063–1071.*

3. **Lesbros-Pantoflickova, D., et al. (2007).** *"Probiotics reduce dysbiosis from acid suppression." Am J Gastroenterol, 102(7), 1531–153*

Printed in Great Britain
by Amazon